TH

PLAC

OF LONDON

STEPHEN PORTER

THE
PLAGUES
OF **LONDON**

TEMPUS

This edition first published 2008

Tempus Publishing
Cirencester Road, Chalford,
Stroud, Gloucestershire, GL6 8PE
www.tempus-publishing.com

Tempus Publishing is an imprint of The History Press Limited

British Library Cataloguing in Publication Data.
A catalogue record for this book is available from the British Library.

ISBN 978 0 7524 4596 0

Typesetting and origination by The History Press Limited
Printed in Great Britain by Ashford Colour Press Ltd., Gosport, Hants.

Contents

About the Author

Stephen Porter, until his recent retirement, worked for over seventeen years for the Survey of London, a century-old project devoted to the history of London's built environment. His other books include *The Great Plague*, *The Great Fire of London*, *London & the Civil War* and *Destruction in the English Civil Wars*. He lives in Stratford-Upon-Avon.

Acknowledgements

Kind invitations from Professor Frank Cox, to give a lecture at Gresham College on plague in early modern London, Alison Bailey, to submit an article on plague for *The Biologist*, and Dr Julian Davies, to speak on the topic of St Giles-in-the-Fields in the Great Plague, helped to focus my thoughts, just at the time when my editor at Tempus, Jonathan Reeve, was persuading me that a book on the subject was needed. I am very grateful to all of them for their encouragement. Kenneth Gage of the Centers for Disease Control and Prevention and Bill White of the Museum of London Archaeology Service kindly gave advice on the aetiology of plague. Gillian Tindall's careful reading of the text and Christabel Scaife's skilful editing saved me from some unnecessary errors and Derek Kendall gave invaluable help with some of the illustrations. My wife Carolyn was good enough to follow my progress and make sound suggestions on the text. The pestilence has taken us from London to Leiden, from Nijmegen to Venice, and she has been startled to discover just how stimulating plague can be.

I

A Most Dreadful Disease

Of all the diseases that afflicted Europe in the pre-modern period, plague made the greatest impact. Devastating and feared, it had a profound effect on the outlook and behaviour of Europeans for more than 400 years after its calamitous onset in the mid-fourteenth century. Its pre-eminence among diseases was such that plague, or 'the pestilence', came to be used to describe not only contagious epidemic diseases but any affliction or calamity, or as a curse upon others: 'A plague on both your houses.'

In King James' Bible of 1611, plague was both a manifestation of God's anger – 'behold, with a great plague will the Lord smite thy people, and thy children, and thy wives, and all thy goods' – and a catastrophe that could strike a city:'The sword is without, and the pestilence and the famine within: he that is in the field shall die with the sword; and he that is in the city, famine and pestilence shall devour him.' It is hardly surprising that this most dreaded of diseases developed a symbolic significance, given the scale of the mortality during the periodic epidemics, and the sheer foulness of the disorder.

The symptoms of bubonic plague included a high fever, headaches, vomiting, the painful swelling of the lymph nodes, especially in the groin and armpits and on the neck, forming the buboes which give the disease its name, and excruciatingly painful blotches or carbuncles up to an inch across, caused by haemorrhaging beneath the skin. These blotches were often described by contemporaries as tokens, and plague as 'spotted death'. The haemorrhaging produced neurological and psychological effects, with the victims often suffering delirium; screaming and running wildly around the streets. The symptoms in themselves and their all too visible effects were enough to produce fear and revulsion. These were intensified by the remorselessness with which plague spread, the speed of death – which generally followed the first appearance of symptoms within a few days, and no longer than a week – and the high fatality rate; Scarrus in Shakespeare's *Antony and Cleopatra* refers to 'the token'd pestilence where death is sure'. This was a (perhaps understandable) exaggeration, for between twenty and thirty per cent of those who contracted the disease survived, usually after their buboes had burst. And they had to burst outwards; if they burst inwards then the victim died of septic shock almost immediately.

Ambrose Barnes was an apprentice to a merchant in Newcastle-upon-Tyne during an outbreak of plague in the late 1640s, and later recalled his awful experience, writing in the third person. The disease 'made for some months an horrible devastation', with the bodies collected at night and taken in carts to be buried outside the city. Eventually, one of the merchant's maids was taken ill, but the other continued to serve meals to Barnes and his master, until Barnes noticed that she was showing 'some dangerous symptoms'. His master left abruptly and took ship for Hamburg; both of the maids died, within a few hours of each other, and Barnes fell ill. He was left alone 'in an empty house… without any living creature besides himself'. Food was placed outside the street door for him to collect. 'In this hideous lonely manner, he spent severall dayes and nights, but God was with him. A huge tumour rose upon his neck behind, the suppuration whereof, physitions were of opinion, saved his life.'

Epidemics of other diseases struck from time to time and some caused high levels of mortality, but plague made the greatest impact on society and was the most feared. In 1603, James Balmford, minister of St Olave's, Southwark, described plague as 'more daungerously contagious being mortall, than the leprosie'. Because of the foulness of the disease and the numbers of its victims his contemporary Thomas Dekker gave plague

> …a Preheminence above all others… none being able to match it, for Violence, Strength, Incertainty, Suttlety, Catching, Universality, and Desolation, it is called the Sicknesse. As if it were, the onely Sicknesse, or the Sicknesse of Sicknesse, as it is indeede.

It has retained its reputation as the deadliest of diseases and is used as a metaphor for disasters or extremely testing circumstances. Discussing the diplomatic exchanges which preceded the Iraq war in 2003, Sir Kieran Prendergast, head of the United Nations' department for Political Affairs, described the Security Council as being faced with a choice between cholera and plague, and commented that 'You always prefer cholera to the plague, because cholera is survivable and the plague much less so'.

The earliest recorded disease bearing a resemblance to plague erupted at Athens in the fifth century BC, but the cause of that epidemic is uncertain. The evolution of the plague bacterium has recently been dated to between 20,000 and 1,500 years ago. Within this long range, the more recent date fits the chronology of the first of the three pandemics, the Plague of Justinian, which struck Egypt in 541 and spread to western Europe in the following year, with periodic epidemics until the 760s. Justinian I was emperor of the eastern Roman Empire and Procopius, secretary to his general, Count Belisarius, described the symptoms of the disease. It began with a fever, which was followed by the eruption of swellings below the abdomen, in the armpit, by the ears and on the thigh, and it produced a deep coma or, in other cases, violent delirium. Those victims whose bodies developed black pustules died shortly afterwards, while those whose tumours burst and discharged pus survived the disease. Justinian himself was infected but lived. The extent of the mortality, an estimated 40 million deaths, can be explained by the impact of this newly evolved bacterium on a population without any specific immunity, induced in response to previous infection, and enfeebled by the effects of several years of disastrous harvests – a result of low levels of sunlight caused by excessive dust in the atmosphere.

The second pandemic was identified in the late 1330s and spread from central Asia to the shores of the Black Sea. In 1345–46 the Genoese were besieged in their colony of Kaffa on the Crimean peninsula by the Tartar army of Kipchak khan Janibeg. When plague broke out among his troops, he shared his misfortune by catapulting the bodies of its victims into the town, where the defenders contracted the disease. According to Gabriele de' Mussi's contemporary account, four Genoese ships broke the blockade and returned to Italy, carrying the disease into the Mediterranean basin. It is improbable that this was the only means by which plague reached Europe, and it may have been dispersed from the Black Sea and eastern Mediterranean along the trade routes, reaching Messina in Sicily in 1347 and, in early 1348, Venice, Pisa, Marseille and Genoa.

The disease, which in the early nineteenth century came to be known as the Black Death, then spread steadily across Europe, probably reaching England in the summer of 1348 and continuing through the following year. In London, the cemeteries were quickly filled and 'very many were compelled to bury their dead in places unseemly and not hallowed or blessed; for some, it was said, cast their corpses into the river'. Extra burial grounds were acquired, one of them at Smithfield, where, according to a papal bull of 1351, more than 60,000 victims were buried, while the foundation charter of the Carthusian priory established on the site in 1371 referred to 50,000 interments there. But London's population before the onset of the plague was no more than 80,000 and perhaps was as low as 45,000 in 1348. The number of burials may have been exaggerated tenfold, or even more.

A society that had undergone the trauma of such an epidemic can hardly be expected to have produced accurate statistics, and no reliance can be placed upon the figures of 23.8 million deaths in Europe, in a pre-plague population of 75 million, produced for Pope Clement VI in 1350. On the other hand, local studies have shown that the proportion of thirty-one per cent, which the figures suggest, may underestimate the scale of the loss in some communities, which experienced an even higher death toll. As in the first pandemic, the impact was that of a 'new disease' on a population which had not been exposed to it before and did not have immunity or the medical knowledge and administrative procedures to contain it.

Further plague epidemics struck western Europe so frequently throughout the late Middle Ages that no genera-tion escaped, and in some outbreaks the proportion of the population that died was as great as during the Black Death. Familiarity with the pattern of such epidemics and awareness of the scale of the mortality did not lessen the grief when death struck. In 1400, Ser Lapo Mazzei wrote from Florence that his family had so far been spared by the outbreak raging in the city, only to have to follow his earlier letters with the news that three of his children had died, two of them within a few hours: 'Imagine how my heart broke... Think of it: three dead!'

The last outbreaks in north-west Europe came in the late seventeenth century, but parts of northern and eastern Europe continued to suffer from plague well into the eighteenth century. The last epidemic in the Mediterranean lands, in Egypt, subsided only in 1835. Although these epidemics did not reach the British Isles, they had an impact through the precautions that were taken, which disrupted trade, and the fear which the disease continued to arouse. Outbreaks in the Baltic lands in 1710 and in southern France in the early 1720s caused great alarm, and a plague panic swept London as late as November 1799, drawing the crisp response that 'several idle rumours respecting the plague are unfounded'.

The third pandemic began in the mid-nineteenth century in central Asia and spread across southern China in 1894. When it reached Hong Kong, Alexandre Yersin and Shibasabuto Kitasato set out separately to isolate the plague bacillus. Yersin succeeded and came to be recognised as the discoverer of the bacillus, which in 1923 was named *Pasteurella pestis*, in acknowledgement of his teacher, Louis Pasteur, and the Pasteur Institute where he had trained. In 1954 it was redesignated *Yersinia pestis*, and that name became adopted internationally in 1980. The means of transmission of the disease were discovered independently by Masanori Ogata in Taiwan and Paul-Louis Simond in Bombay. Even when this had been understood and, for the first time, countermeasures could be targeted at the cause, plague continued to claim many victims, with

12.6 million people dying of the disease in India between 1898 and 1948.

As observed during the third pandemic, the plague bacillus is transmitted by the bite of a rat's flea, *Xenopsylla cheopis*. The flea's mouth sucks blood from its host, and also squirts saliva containing partly digested blood into the bite. As the flea feeds on the blood of its infected host, the ingested bacilli multiply to such an extent that they block the proventriculus, the organ at the entrance to the flea's stomach. When the rat dies and the flea transfers to a human and attempts to feed, the passage of blood into its stomach is obstructed by the blocked proventriculus. Unable to ingest the blood, the flea becomes ravenous and continues to feed, to the point where the blood is regurgitated with the saliva, carrying the plague bacilli into the bite in the skin of its human host. The flea starves to death.

Septicaemic plague is also caused by a flea bite, but the bacilli enter the bloodstream directly, not through the lymphatic system, resulting in a more rapid death than with the victims of bubonic plague, and before buboes have formed. Pneumonic plague develops when the bacterium enters the lungs, with respiratory droplets the means of direct transmission from person to person, requiring close contact with a victim. Both septicaemic and pneumonic plague are much less common than the bubonic form, but have a fatality rate of 100 per cent when untreated.

An average of 1,700 cases of plague a year were reported to the World Health Organisation during the second half of the twentieth century, and *Yersinia pestis* occurs in rodents in every continent except Europe. The mortality rate has fallen sharply with the development of antibiotics – streptomycin, gentamicin and tetracycline – but nevertheless remains high in small outbreaks where diagnosis and treatment are slow. During an outbreak in Uganda in October 2001, there were fourteen fatalities from twenty-three reported cases, and in February

2002 four people died and another twelve were infected in a village in the Indian state of Himachal Pradesh. By comparison, during the outbreak of Severe Acute Respiratory Syndrome (SARS) in 2003 the fatality rate was below ten per cent.

Analysis of the genetic structure of *Yersinia pestis* has shown that it evolved from *Yersinia pseudotuberculosis* and that there is little genetic difference between the two. Yet *Y. pseudotuberculosis* causes gut infections and *Y. pestis* has been a major scourge of mankind for much of the past 1,500 years. Three sub-types of *Y. pestis* have been distinguished, each associated with one of the plague pandemics and originating in different parts of the world. The Plague of Justinian was caused by the sub-type Antiqua, the second pandemic by Mediaevalis and the third by Orientalis. They originated in central and east Africa, Kurdistan, and the Yunnan region of China, respectively.

The responses to the medieval plagues were produced by a society which was wholly ignorant of the cause of the disease and struggled to deal with its effects. The descriptions which were generated have to be interpreted in the light of modern knowledge and more than a century of observation of cases during the third pandemic. For example, contemporary references to the fetid breath of the victims and their coughing up of bloody sputum have led to the suggestion that pneumonic plague was an element in the spread of the Black Death. It would explain the continuing virulence of the disease throughout the winter months, as people spent more time indoors gathered around fires and stoves and so had closer contact than during the summer. But winter deaths are not a sure indication of pneumonic plague and that pattern was not replicated in the epidemics in the sixteenth and seventeenth centuries, when mortality during the winter was very much lower than in the summer and early autumn.

The quantity and quality of evidence increased throughout the long period of the second pandemic, as governments expanded their authority, more records were created and more survived. The seasonality of the disease can be determined from burial registers, many of which distinguish plague deaths. They show two chronologies for plague epidemics. In one of them, the disease appeared in the spring and increased during June and July, to peak in August or early September. In the second, the outbreak began in the summer and peaked in the autumn. During the sixteenth century, a procedure was devised for the examination of the symptoms on the patient or body in order to identify the disease. Plague was distinguishable from fevers, and when 'the tokens, tumors, or carbuncle do appeare, there is no cause of suspition or doubt of the disease'.

The wider pattern suggests that the environment in north-west Europe during the second pandemic was too cool to maintain active foci of infection, and that the disease was not endemic, requiring periodic re-infection. Plague was a disease of the trade routes, both international and internal, with the eastern Mediterranean the region from which it spread over the continent, albeit erratically. The epidemics in early modern London support the notion of new infections, with an outbreak beginning in some districts and spreading from them, rather than erupting across the city more or less simultaneously, as the conditions for the disease became favourable. And they followed epidemics in Antwerp and Amsterdam, the principal cities trading with London.

Even so, the speed with which such epidemics developed, within a few weeks, the high mortality rates and the absence of references to dead rats in large numbers during plague outbreaks have led to doubts about the role of rats and their fleas in the diffusion of the disease. Dead and dying rats were noticed during epidemics in China in the late eighteenth century and were a conspicuous aspect of the outbreaks of bubonic plague in China and India in the 1890s. But they were not mentioned in epidemics in early modern London, even though

they did not escape attention as a possible cause of the spread
of the disease, together with stray dogs and cats. Fleas were also
noticed in connection with plague. In 1625, Stephen Bradwell
noted that tokens were spots, 'of the bignesse of Flea-bitings'
or larger, but a direct connection between fleas and the disease
was not made.

The failure to mention the deaths of rats was not because they
were not present. By the sixteenth century they had become
a pest in towns and cities, living in association with humans
and their livestock, in barns and housing. The Carthusian
monks were vegetarian, but had a meat kitchen where meals
for their guests were prepared. At their London priory, in 1500
they found it necessary to install hangings for beef and bacon
suspended from the kitchen roof 'for defence against ratts'. A
century later, Simon Forman, in Lambeth, was less careful, and
rats ate his pigeons; at the time of the Great Plague in 1665
Sir Robert Long told his clerk at his house in New Palace
Yard, Westminster, to 'take all course you can agaynst the ratts'.
Rats and mice were so successful at colonising rural areas, as
well as towns, that in the mid-seventeenth century they were
described as pests whose depredations were familiar to almost
everyone living in the countryside.

Rats are agile, resourceful and prolific. A female has between
five and ten pups in a litter, which can be weaned after three
weeks and are able to breed when they are twelve weeks old.
Even though the mobility of individual rats is limited, a rat
population supports large numbers of fleas, especially when
they are too ill to groom efficiently. A rat flea can jump 200
times its own length (typically one-tenth of an inch) and
130 times its height. *Xenopsylla cheopis* is the principal flea
parasite of the black rat, *rattus rattus*, but observations during
the third pandemic have shown that both brown and black
rats are the hosts of infective fleas. Epidemics erupt when the
host rat population reaches a critical density. This has been

demonstrated by a study of gerbil burrows in central Asia, which are reservoirs of plague; *Y. pestis* appeared roughly two years after the occupation of the burrows began to increase significantly.

The human flea, *Pulex irritans*, may also have been a carrier once the disease had been introduced and an epidemic was under way. It is capable of being infected with *Y. pestis* and among its wide range of hosts are domesticated animals, including dogs, cats and pigs. Laboratory tests suggest that to transmit the disease *P. irritans* must be present in large numbers, bite a host carrying many bacteria and quickly pass the infection to another host. When these conditions are met, *Y. pestis* can be transferred by the human flea, with plague spreading quickly, and social and economic contacts influencing the diffusion of the disease.

The fleas require relatively high temperatures and humidity; essentially, the greater the humidity the lower the temperature at which it can survive, but the ideal conditions are ninety to ninety-five per cent humidity and temperatures of fifteen to twenty-five degrees centigrade. In such microclimates as those provided by a rat's nest or stocks of grain, which hold residuary heat beyond the peak temperatures of the summer months, fleas can live for up to a year, and they have some tolerance to cold weather in the context of mammals' burrows. Cases of direct human plague infection from animals in Colorado in December 1983, and Washington state and Texas in January 1984, indicate that plague deaths noted during winter in the historical record should not be dismissed as contemporary misidentification of the disease. The microclimate provided by a rat's nest in an urban environment should have been sufficiently warm for fleas to survive and would have allowed contact with humans. Fleas can carry the infection through the winter months and some wild rodents can become infected prior to hibernation and develop plague when they awaken in the spring. Rat and flea populations may be reduced by harsh winters, but they recover quickly.

From the isolation of the plague bacillus in the 1890s, the bubonic plague of the third pandemic has been equated with the causative disease of the first two pandemics. Yet in some ways its characteristics, especially as observed by the Indian Plague Commission, differ from those reported or identified in Europe between the fourteenth and eighteenth centuries. Some allowance has to be made for the different impact of *Y. pestis medievalis* in a temperate maritime climate and *Y. pestis orientalis* in a sub-tropical one. Even so, there have been doubts about the nature of the disease, with anthrax, typhus and tuberculosis suggested as possible contributory diseases to plague epidemics.

A more radical proposition is that the causative agent was not a bacterium but a haemorrhagic virus, supposed to be a filovirus similar to the Ebola or Marburg viruses. According to this hypothesis, bubonic plague was present in the Mediterranean basin but not in northern Europe or the British Isles, where the epidemics were of a haemorrhagic fever. Rashes are among the symptoms of the Ebola virus, but they appear within a few days of infection, and with Marburg haemorrhagic fever after an incubation period of five to ten days. Rashes could be similar to the tokens characteristic of bubonic plague, but could not be confused with buboes. The symptoms of the epidemic fevers which erupted in the eighteenth century included carbuncles, but contemporaries did not equate them with plague buboes, nor did they regard the diseases as plague, although they were still very much alert to the possibility of a plague epidemic.

A DNA-detection technique devised during the 1990s, known as suicide PCR, has raised the possibility that *Y. pestis* can be identified from archaeological material from the second pandemic. The problem of subsequent contamination has been a confounding factor for analysis of material from sites such as cesspits or burial grounds, but this is overcome by applying the technique to dental pulp, which is durable, likely to harbour infection and free from external contamination. Tests on the DNA from dental pulp of unerupted teeth, from skulls in plague burial grounds in southern France, including some that were interred during the Black Death, revealed the presence of *Y. pestis*, while the pulp from non-plague burials did not contain traces of the bacterium. However, the results of those tests have not been replicated elsewhere; *Y. pestis* is a delicate microorganism and detectable traces may have vanished since the epidemics of the second pandemic.

Whatever the disease and the means of transmission, contemporaries could deal with outbreaks only within the framework of their medical knowledge. This was based largely upon the writings of the Classical authors, especially the Greek physician Hippocrates, who lived during the fifth century BC, and the interpretation of their ideas by Galen, a court physician in second-century Rome. Galen believed that disease resulted from an imbalance of the four humours in the body: blood, phlegm, choler and melancholy. Such an imbalance was caused by the corruption of the air from 'a putrid exhalation' produced by rotting matter and, during the summer months, emissions from stagnant water, such as that in marshes and ponds. These harmful miasmas were the result of a particular conjunction of the planets. An individual's health was affected by the planets and signs of the zodiac, for each planet was believed to influence a part of the body and their arrangement therefore determined a person's well-being. A doctor needed to know his patient's exact time and place of birth before proceeding to diagnosis and treatment, which often involved the letting of a specified quantity of blood. Contagion was not part of Classical medical theory, yet the term was used during the Black Death and subsequent outbreaks, and the disease was thought to spread through contact, infecting those who had touched its victims or their belongings.

The connection between miasma and plague was made soon after the Black Death first struck London, in a letter from Edward III to the Lord Mayor complaining of the poisoned air caused by the pollution of public places, and again during the epidemic in 1361, when the king objected to the stench caused by the slaughter of animals within the city. Contaminated air was associated with diseases. By the sixteenth century both miasma and contagion provided explanations for illness. Sir Thomas More's *Utopia* of 1516 explained his ideal, that nothing 'filthy, loathsome, or uncleanly be brought into the city, lest the air, by the stench thereof infected and corrupt, should cause pestilent disease'. This clear statement of the risk of miasmic air is followed by the care taken to prevent the transmission of disease in the hospital, where the sick were not placed close together, so that those 'taken and holden with contagious diseases, such as be wont by infection to creep from one to another, might be laid apart from the company of the residue'. Disease could be transmitted from person to person and the danger was greater in miasmic air. A Veronese physician, Gerolamo Fracastoro, gave contagion a theoretical basis in 1546 with the publication of his *De Contagione*, in which he described three means of contagion: by contact, by carriers such as clothes, and by *seminaria*, which can move, propagate and die.

The measures gradually adopted to combat plague during the late Middle Ages by governments, national and local, reflected anxieties concerning both foul air and contagion. Some were designed to prevent clean and wholesome air being turned into tainted air by removing putrid and offensively smelly matter, such as offal and manure, and by the cleansing or draining of ditches and pools. Others attempted to prevent potentially dangerous contacts. Incoming travellers and cargoes were halted outside a town, with goods, especially textiles, fumigated or left open to the air. The period of detention was commonly forty days, hence the term quarantine. Cordons were put in place outside a town and, by the early sixteenth century, travellers coming from an area known, or even suspected, to be suffering from plague were admitted only on the production of a pass stating that they had not been anywhere the disease was active. Those within the community who were suffering from plague were removed to isolation hospitals, known as pesthouses, for segregation and treatment. If no spaces were available – during an epidemic the pesthouses were hopelessly inadequate – the sick and those who had been in contact with them were detained in their houses. Information gathering was improved, and from the growing numbers of plague victims the onset of an outbreak could be recognised at an early stage, enabling cordons, quarantines and other measures to be put in place.

The Italian states were in the forefront in adopting such public health procedures and developing the administrative organisation to implement them. But implementation was not invariably straightforward, for the policies were economically and socially disruptive at the level of both communities and households and met with resistance or evasion by the population they were intended to safeguard. Even so, they provided the pattern for controls introduced elsewhere across Europe and may have prevented some epidemics, but, despite such successes and the advantages to public health and hygiene, large-scale outbreaks of plague continued to erupt periodically.

Without any completely effective prevention of the outbreaks, or satisfactory explanations for them, plague was seen, with famine and war, as one of God's three mortal arrows, which he could unleash to punish sinners or send as warnings to repent. An epidemic did seem to resemble the effect of a cloud of arrows fired into a crowd, killing some at random and leaving others untouched. It provided an opportunity for the clergy and moral writers to condemn the population for its woeful behaviour and plead for repentance and reform, so that God would relent and end the plague. Expiatory services and penitential processions were held, and the saints were beseeched to intercede, so that the community would be spared before being completely wiped out. Some saints were especially venerated for their influence in times of plague. Saint Sebastian had survived being pierced by arrows, which inflicted the sharp pain characteristic of the disease, only to be pummelled to death, and Saint Roch, a hermit, had been succoured by a dog when he caught the plague and so had survived. Artists commonly depicted Saint Sebastian wounded by pestilent arrows, saving others who could have been the victims, but those who painted Saint Roch, such as the fifteenth-century Venetian Carlo Crivelli, made a more direct reference to the plague by showing him with a large bubo on his thigh.

Services and processions were potential sources of friction between the clergy and the civil authorities, who disapproved of people gathering together in case the disease was spread further. The clergy could point out that none of the measures taken were effective and that the plague would be halted only through the intercession of the saints. Their claims seemed to be justified when epidemics subsided, and in Counter-Reformation Europe, gratitude for the ending of the plague was expressed in the commissioning of works of art, the construction of churches – such as the Redentore and Santa Maria della Salute in Venice – and, in the Austrian empire after the plague of 1679, the erection of plague columns.

Protestant Europe abandoned appeals to the saints, but did hold special services and observe fast days. William Tyndale ridiculed those who followed a routine of fasting on Thursdays for a part of the year, 'and that to be delivered of the pestilence'.

In 1630, Roman Catholic entreaties to Saint Sebastian were also questioned in rational terms: 'If it lieth not in the power of mortal men that are living with us to helpe, how much lesse can they that are dead? And farre lesse, one that perhaps hath never beene.' But this denial of the efficacy of saints fell short of questioning the existence of a wrathful God, regarded as the source of plague and prayed to for respite. The Anglican liturgy incorporated prayers for deliverance from the plague, with fast days stipulated during epidemics, and included in the Litany the entreaty: 'From lightning and tempest; from plague, pestilence, and famine; from battle and murder, and from sudden death, good Lord, deliver us.'

Providentialist interpretations by the clergy and moralists did not lead to passive acceptance by a populace faced with periodic outbreaks of death on a large scale. The cause and remedy of plague were regarded as both supernatural and natural, and a whole host of preventative medicines were recommended, and a cure earnestly wished for. When Christopher Marlowe's Dr Faustus considered how best to use his talents, he imagined his prescriptions 'hung up as monuments, whereby whole cities have escaped the plague'. Marlowe's point was that this would indeed have been a major contribution to the well-being of mankind and would have given Faustus a kind of immortality. Ben Jonson mocked those who professed to have devised preventatives for the plague, through the character of Sir Epicure Mammon in *The Alchemist*, who claims to have developed a medicine which can not only reverse the ageing process, but also 'fright the plague out o'the kingdome in three months'.

In reality, many suggestions were offered, some designed to gain immunity by keeping the air sweet and warding off the noxious fumes with strong smells. Herbs were popular, with rosemary, rue, lavender, sage, mint and wormwood especially favoured, as embrocations and as the fillings for nosegays and

pomanders, and the nutmeg came to be highly prized for the
contents of pomanders, some of which were so finely made
that they were as much fashion accessories as guards against
plague. Householders would place bunches of fragrant herbs at
their doors and windows to ensure that only pure air wafted
into their houses.

The smells did not have to be sweet; any strong odour might
serve the purpose. Smoking or chewing tobacco was thought to
bring immunity, and in 1665 Dr Francis Glisson recommended
as his 'constant antidote' a piece of dried manure of someone
who had died of the disease, kept in a house in a porous box
for 'the best antidotical perfume'. After a diplomatic mission to
Spain in the 1660s, the Earl of Sandwich recalled that Madrid,
where it was the practice for the householders to throw their
excrement into the streets, was 'the stinkingst town they ever
came into', a characteristic which the Madrileños long believed
gave their city protection against plague. Advice provided by Sir
Theodore de Mayerne and Thomas Cademan appealed to taste
rather than smell, with a recipe for a plague water that consisted
of three pints of muscadine wine, mixed with sage, rue, ginger,
nutmeg, pepper and treacle, with the assurance that: 'All the
Plague time... trust to this, for there was never man, woman, or
childe, that failed of their expectation in taking of it.'

This was not the advice of charlatans or eccentrics. Glisson
was Regius Professor of Physic at Cambridge for more than
forty years, a Fellow of the College of Physicians and an original fellow of the Royal Society, and de Mayerne and Cademan
were physicians to Charles I and Henrietta Maria. That such
distinguished men should give such fatuous advice is indicative
of how ineffectual a whole range of supposed preventatives had
been, after more than 300 years' experience of the disease. Had
a credible antidote or remedy been found, there would have
been no market for the new ideas and variations on old ones
that continued to be recommended and tried.

If foul air could not be repelled by sweet or sour air, perhaps it could be absorbed. *Present Remedies against the Plague*, published in 1594, claimed that three or four peeled onions left on the ground for ten days would absorb all the infection in the neighbourhood. This, too, was an eccentric solution. A more generally accepted notion was that circulation of the air would prevent it stagnating and turning foul, and so householders lit fires and even discharged firearms in their rooms to circulate the air. In attempting to reduce the risk of plague, they increased the danger of a conflagration, which was further enhanced by the practice of lighting bonfires in the streets.

Whatever steps were taken by the civil authorities or clergy, from the first appearance of the disease in Europe in the mid-fourteenth century safety was seen to lie not in precautionary measures or medicines, but in flight. During the Black Death, Gabriele de' Mussi summarised the dilemma: 'Lamenting our misery, we feared to fly, yet we dared not remain.' Writing from London in 1454, William Paston was in no doubt about the action that he should take: 'Here is great pestilence. I purpose to flee into the country.' In 1490, Edward Plumpton, an attorney, reacted in the same way, but added a phrase to justify his decision: 'Sir, they begin to die in London, & then I must departe for the tyme & other men do.'

Those who could go did so, as soon as possible. They had to leave their houses and businesses, perhaps in the care of servants or apprentices, and possibly a prey to burglars, and find a refuge with tenants, business contacts, friends or relatives elsewhere, meeting suspicion and hostility in the process as possible carriers of the dreaded disease. Inevitably, the wealthier citizens not tied to their business or trade were those who could go, while the poorer ones had to remain and take their chances. Some faced harassment as well as the plague. The fear and foreboding produced by an epidemic generated suspicion of groups on the fringes of society, such as beggars, vagrants and foreigners, who were seen as potential threats and were driven out or harshly treated. In parts of medieval Europe, outbreaks of plague were accompanied by persecution of the Jews.

Rulers and the apparatus of state left, and kept on the move if plague broke out wherever they had settled. Government had to continue, whatever the misery that a capital city was enduring; the chaos that would ensue if the political leadership succumbed would help neither city nor nation. But what of those who could make a difference, practical or palliative, especially the magistrates, physicians, apothecaries and clergy? Should they stay, aware that there was little or nothing that they could do to stop the epidemic, or save themselves and return to help the re-establishment of normal life when the outbreak had subsided? This created a fundamental moral dilemma, a choice between the strong probability of death and the likelihood of further life. It had a practical side, too, for it was quite possible that those physicians and clergy who chose not to stay during an epidemic would provoke bitterness and condemnation as runaways in the communities to which they would return. The physicians' typical response was that they had to look after their clients, and that when they had left there was no point in the physicians staying. Of course, not all members of the medical profession left, and some stayed behind so that they could treat the victims in the pesthouses. But the general reaction at times of plague was resentment of those who had gone, rather than appreciation of those who remained.

Others, too, provoked bitterness for abandoning their responsibilities to their family and household, street and neighbourhood. By leaving, they withdrew not only practical help but also financial aid for those affected by the epidemic. This made the efforts of those attempting to implement regulations and tackle the effects of the pestilence more difficult, for resources were reduced at a time of increasing need, and the resentment of those who were compelled to remain when

their social superiors had gone spilled over into defiance of
authority and even disorder. While the poor attracted sympathy as the most numerous victims of plague, bearing the
brunt of epidemics, they were also feared, as the harbourers
of infection who no longer needed to respect authority and
whose indignation and anger might even lead to deliberate
attempts to spread the disease.

Protestant theologians addressed the morality of fleeing
when plague threatened. While accepting the sense of taking
such a precaution, they generally agreed that some members of
the community should remain, including magistrates and clergy,
and anyone who could care for members of their family and
neighbours – categories which included the greater part of the
population. One of Martin Luther's arguments for congregations contributing to the maintenance of their pastors was that
the pastors would visit them during plagues, at considerable
personal risk. In 1537, Miles Coverdale translated for English
readers a tract by the Lutheran theologian Andreas Osiander,
entitled *How and whither a Christen man ought to flye the horrible
Plage*. Despite its title, this did not resolve the dilemma, for
while Osiander did not seek to forbid anyone from moving
away to avoid dangerous places, he wrote that they should not
do so against God's commandment, their calling or love of
their neighbours. Victims died alone because of the 'childish
fear' of those who would not care for them. God's teaching and
duty obliged them to stay. John Hooper, Bishop of Worcester
and Gloucester, wrote in 1553 that clergymen who left their
congregations during plague were 'hirelings and no pastors'.
He, too, held that those in administrative and legal positions
should stay, and recognised that, even though the safest course
was to leave and escape the corrupt air, the poor could not do
so because they had 'no friends nor place to flee unto'.

The moral obligation was undeniable, yet fear was the over-
riding motivation. Thomas Vincent explained that plague was

'very terrible' to those who contracted it, because of the great probability of death, and also to those who did not have it, who were afraid of being infected. This 'razed out of their hearts, for the while, all affections of love and pity to their nearest and dearest friends', who were abandoned as soon as the disease was recognised. Desiderius Erasmus was almost neurotically anxious about plague and when, in 1513, he was in London during an epidemic, he decided not to return to his lodgings to collect his belongings. Subsequently, he changed his mind and 'in complete solitude' went to his room to pack his books and other possessions for collection, and then 'I hurried away and never even slept in my room'.

Erasmus was afraid of being in London during outbreaks of plague, partly because 'I am quite out of sympathy with this nation's dirty habits, habits with which I am already well enough acquainted'. He was especially critical of the English practice of covering the floors of rooms with rushes, which were added to rather than replaced, so that the bottom layer remained for years, impregnated with 'spittle, vomit, the urine of dogs and men, the dregs of beer, the remains of fish, and other nameless filth'. The cumulative effect of such woeful household hygiene, and the use of public places such as the city ditches for depositing 'much filth', prompted Sir Philip Hoby in 1557 to characterise London as 'a stinking city, the filthiest of the world'. The many cesspits within the city and the disposal of rubbish in the ditches, streams and the Thames itself no doubt contributed to the malodorous quality noted by Sir Philip. But public hygiene was not neglected. The streets were cleaned by scavengers and rakers, and the refuse was removed in dung boats or taken away to manure the gardens and fields around the city. Fines were imposed on those who broke the regulations, for example by polluting common water-courses or dumping manure and other rubbish in the streets.

The medieval city was adequately supplied with water, from the Thames and its tributaries, wells and an increasing number of aqueducts that brought fresh water into the centre. In the mid-thirteenth century, a system was laid carrying water from springs near Tyburn to a conduit in Cheapside, and the system was extended during the fifteenth century. New public conduits and cisterns were built from time to time from charitable donations by citizens – there were eleven cisterns by 1500 – and many of London's monasteries had their own supplies. The Greyfriars at Newgate was supplied with piped water from the mid-thirteenth century, and St John's and St Mary's, in Clerkenwell, and St Bartholomew's were all provided with piped water before the early 1430s, when an aqueduct was built connecting springs at Islington with the Charterhouse. The unused water was tapped by the occupiers of houses and inns near the priory, and so the system, which remained in use until the middle of the eighteenth century, served the neighbourhood as well as the monastic community. Wells were sunk within individual premises and a parish well was maintained by many of the vestries, who converted them to pumps during the sixteenth century, reducing both contamination and the risk of accidents to adventurous children.

London did have a high mortality rate in non-plague years, a result of its economic role as well as living conditions, and suffered repeated plague epidemics during the late Middle Ages, with eleven outbreaks between 1407 and 1479. Yet by the beginning of the sixteenth century it had roughly 50,000 inhabitants, a figure which was maintained by a large and steady influx of new arrivals, which partly compensated for the excess of deaths over births and partly replaced those who had returned to their communities after a spell in London. It drew migrants from the remainder of the country because of its role and status as the national capital and by far the largest and wealthiest city. A Venetian envoy in 1500 described it as 'truly the metropolis of England', attracting people from 'all parts of the island, and from Flanders, and from every other place'. The many newcomers to London encountered a cock-tail of diseases to which they had little or no immunity, and the city's internal, coastal and overseas trading links ensured a steady replenishment of the cocktail.

The English were 'great lovers of themselves, and of every-thing belonging to them'. And so it was not surprising that they had 'an antipathy to foreigners, and imagine that they never come into their island, but to make themselves mas-ters of it, and to usurp their goods'. Nevertheless, London's population included perhaps as many as 3,000 aliens, mainly from the Low Countries and France. By the mid-fifteenth century the lands around the North Sea had developed into an economic and cultural region, with London as one of its principal ports. It had grown to be one of the largest cities of north-west Europe by the early sixteenth century, rivalling its major trading partners. Paris was much larger, but London was slightly more populous than Antwerp and considerably bigger than Bruges, which had a population of 30,000, and Amsterdam, which was only a quarter of the size of London at that date.

London's position at the lowest bridging point of the Thames and in the wealthiest and most densely populated part of England gave it strong advantages, as a trading city and the national capital. The Venetian envoy reported that it abounded 'with every article of luxury, as well as with the necessaries of life' and that its 'great riches' derived not from the presence of members of the aristocracy and gentry, but from the com-mercial activities of the merchants and 'persons of low degree'. London's economic success in the late Middle Ages was partly based on its increasing share of overseas trade, especially of woollen cloth, England's most valuable export. In the late four-teenth century London accounted for no more than thirty per cent of cloth exports, but by the early sixteenth century the proportion was seventy per cent, and continuing to rise. The same pattern occurred in other branches of trade, both exports and imports, and by the sixteenth century the port of London handled between seventy and eighty per cent of overseas commerce. Much of the cloth went to Antwerp, but some was processed in London, either for export or for the inland trade, and the capital was important for its manufacturing sector, as well as its role as a distributive centre, especially of wine and other imported goods. It provided, in itself, a large and affluent market for high-value commodities, and for foodstuffs and fuel that were drawn from a considerable area of south-east England and ports along the east coast.

In the 1520s, London contained no more than three per cent of the national population, yet tax assessments suggest that it generated at least twelve per cent of the lay wealth and ten times that produced by Norwich, the next largest English city. London's riches were unevenly distributed, with eighty per cent of those rated for the tax of 1522, known as 'the Loan', valued at below £5 each and together holding just 7.2 per cent of the total, while the wealthiest eighty-seven citizens, fewer than one per cent, were taxed at more than £500 and held 41.7 per cent of the city's wealth. If poverty could be equated with vulnerability to plague, as contemporaries believed, then many of London's citizens were at risk during an epidemic.

The taxation figures were for the administrative city of London, on the north side of the Thames and occupying a slightly larger area than that enclosed within the medieval walls. Conveniently referred to as 'the City', it contained not only the wealthiest merchants and tradesmen, but also more than a score of religious houses. Roughly a quarter of those who plied their trade in the City were freemen – a status acquired by apprenticeship, patrimony, or a fee – which conferred political and economic rights. They were organised into livery companies, or guilds, which regulated the trades and crafts. For civil administration, the City was divided into twenty-five wards until 1550, when the area at the south end of London Bridge became the twenty-sixth, and there were 113 parishes. The City was ruled by a council of aldermen, one for each ward, with one of them serving as Lord Mayor for a year, and a much larger but less powerful Common Council of more than 200 members, elected through the wards. The jurisdictions of wards and parish vestries overlapped to some extent, and their officers oversaw a variety of matters, including the enforcement of environmental regulations. The wards, parishes and livery companies also shared the responsibility for implementing orders imposed by the government and the Lord Mayor and aldermen.

The suburbs on the north side of the river, which were beginning to expand beyond the area within the corporation's control, were governed by the Middlesex justices of the peace. That to the west, beyond the legal quarter and the bishops' palaces lining the Strand, linked London to Westminster, with its abbey of St Peter and the royal palace. Because of its low-lying site and the miasmas emanating from nearby marshy ground, Westminster was thought to be particularly susceptible to plague. On the south side of the Thames, across the only bridge, was the substantial but somewhat disreputable suburb of Southwark, which contained the houses of bishops and abbots, and inns catering for travellers coming to the city from the south, but also alehouses and brothels. The suburbs south of the river were administered by the Surrey justices.

Between 1536 and 1542, London's monastic houses were dissolved. Some were converted into aristocratic mansions, but the process was slow enough for the Venetian ambassador to note in 1554 that the city was still 'much disfigured by the ruins of a multitude of churches and monasteries'. The dissolution was not a check to London's prosperity, however, and may indeed have been a spur to growth. Not only did the extensive property of the London monasteries become available for development, so too did the London properties of more than 100 other religious houses around the country. In addition, some of the bishops' London houses were forcibly appropriated, so that the Strand became lined with aristocratic, not ecclesiastical, mansions. The scars were healed by new building, as the former monastic sites were redeveloped to house the expanding population. While the great houses of the aristocracy and prelates were of stone, new building in the sixteenth century was in brick, although the bulk of the houses were timber-framed, with lath and plaster infilling, standing several storeys high in the principal streets. In the alleys behind were smaller, insubstantial timber cottages, many of which contained only one room. Wood predominated to such an extent that James I described London as a 'Citie... of Stickes'.

By the end of the fifteenth century, London was preeminent as the political, legal and economic capital of England and was the largest and wealthiest city within the British Isles. But its very size and extensive functions made it susceptible to epidemic diseases, including plague. This continued to strike periodically, despite increasing attempts from the early sixteenth century, by central and local government, to prevent its occurrence and limit its effects if it did gain a foothold in the city. The measures adopted, and the response to them by the citizens of Tudor and Stuart London, contributed to the impact of plague, which was the most socially divisive and economically disruptive of all diseases.

2

Plague and Precept in Tudor London

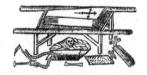

With Richard III's defeat at the battle of Bosworth in August 1485, Plantagenet rule came to an end. His conqueror, Henry Tudor, took the throne as Henry VII, founding a new, albeit fragile, dynasty which was to last for only three generations. Rebellions were suppressed and pretenders defeated or isolated diplomatically, but premature deaths and failure to produce heirs caused great concern, as well as emphasising the need to protect the monarch from disease. Isolation was not desirable, for the monarch had to be accessible and available to conduct business and preside at court. During epidemics, the normal arrangements were

modified and the court avoided infected places, which generally included London, but when the danger was perceived to
be very great, it broke up altogether.

Bosworth was followed by the appearance of a new and
deadly disease, perhaps transmitted by Henry's troops, and
1485 was remembered as the year with 'a gret dethe and
hasty, called swettyng syknes'. Polydore Vergil described the
sweat, which came to be known as the English Sweat (*Sudor
Anglicus*), as a disease 'which no previous age had experienced', that swept across the whole country. Probably a viral
infection, it seems to have been introduced into a population
which had no immunity, producing a level of mortality so
high that it was said that 'scarcely one in a hundred' of those
who contracted the disease survived. Death generally came
within twenty-four hours, so that a victim could have been
'merry at dinner and dead at supper', and it struck the well-
nourished as well as the poor, carrying off noblemen and
courtiers. Those who survived did not then have immunity,
but were liable to suffer repeated attacks. Experience showed
that the best treatment was to go to bed fully clothed and
wrap up under the bedclothes, lying still for twenty-four
hours, taking warm drinks, but eating nothing and not exposing so much as an arm to the air.

The sweat caused great alarm and a 'disastrous loss of life',
but plague remained the greatest danger and the largest killer.
The scale of an epidemic, and whether the numbers of victims
were increasing or decreasing, were assessed from reports from
the infected areas. Collection of statistics of plague deaths to
provide reliable evidence, which had been introduced by some
Italian cities in the fifteenth century, had not yet been adopted
in England. Indeed, English authorities, both central and local,
were distinctly sluggish in attempting to tackle the plague
and the sweating sickness, compared not only with the Italian
states, but also with much of northern Europe.

The close of the fifteenth century was a sickly time in London. An epidemic struck in 1498 and continued until 1500, affecting many places, 'but most of all in the citie of London, where died in that yeare thirtie thousand'. A more realistic assessment is that 10,000 died in that outbreak, or roughly twenty per cent of the population. The sweat returned in 1508–09 and epidemics of both the sweat and plague occurred intermittently during the 1510s and 1520s. In 1513, 'the great plague' continued in London from the spring until the autumn, with the death toll in October still as high as between 300 and 400 each day, a figure which, if accurate and sustained, suggests a severe outbreak. In an epidemic two years later, twenty-seven nuns of the Poor Clares and some of their servants died of the plague in their house at the Minories, which did not prove to be a refuge once the infection had penetrated into the community.

Henry VIII had come to the throne on his father's death in 1509, having married his brother Arthur's widow, Catherine of Aragon. Mary, born in 1516, was the only one of their children to survive infancy. Following Henry's divorce from Catherine and marriage to Anne Boleyn, a second daughter, Elizabeth, was born in 1533, but only after a third marriage, to Jane Seymour, did the king have a male heir, with the birth of Prince Edward in 1537. For much of his reign, Henry was extremely concerned to escape any dangerous disease which might kill him before he had secured the Tudor dynasty by producing a son.

The king was, therefore, most anxious when the sweat returned in July 1517. The outbreak 'carried many off', prompting Sir Thomas More to comment that there was less danger on the battlefield than in London. Plague followed the sweat, continuing through the autumn. No steps had yet been taken to attempt to check the spread of the disease in London or elsewhere, although the rules for the court codified under Edward IV included the stipulation that 'There ought no perilous sykeman to lodge in this courte, but to avoyde within three dayes'. But the safest course during an epidemic was for the court to move away from all infected places, rather than simply expel those who were sick. In 1517 it withdrew, at first to Windsor, but the king's anxiety was heightened by the deaths of courtiers such as Lords Clinton and Grey, as well as 'many other knights and gentlemen', and, more immediately, two pages in the royal household. He then took the extreme step of dismissing virtually everyone, retaining only a few gentlemen to attend upon himself and the queen, and he went to an undisclosed 'remote and unusual habitation', where he withdrew from 'all business'. This was really rather ridiculous. The king was noted for his physical courage and was prepared to take on all challengers in the jousts, yet the threat of plague caused him not just to move to a palace outside London where access could be controlled, but to isolate himself somewhere in the countryside of the Thames valley.

His anxiety explains why the court did not return to London in the winter, when the epidemic had died down, and Cardinal Thomas Wolsey, the Lord Chancellor since 1515, had come back. But the prolonged absence of the court and the failure to keep Christmas, when the citizens were permitted to come and watch the festivities, caused 'general discontent' in the capital. The absence of the court had an economic impact on those who supplied it with food and drink, horses and livery, clothes and luxury goods. Its continued absence was injurious and likely to prove unpopular. A hostile capital is a potential threat to any government, acting as the focus of political opposition and liable to erupt if the citizens' antagonism cannot be assuaged, as Charles I was to discover. Wolsey was unwilling to overlook the rumbling discontent and, no doubt mindful of the xenophobic and murderous Evil May Day riots in 1517, ordered the City authorities to seek out those who uttered 'seditious words' against the king for leaving London.

Wolsey also set out to tackle the causes of the dissemination as well as the consequences of the disease which so alarmed the king – and periodically devastated the capital's population – by introducing, in January 1518, the first measures in England aimed at reducing the incidence of plague. A royal proclamation declared that the 'resorting of persons not infected with the pestilence to other persons infected doth daily cause the increase of further infection, to the great mortality and death of many persons which, by reason of such resort one to another, have been ignorantly infected with the said pestilence'. To limit such contacts, it required that any house in London which contained someone infected with plague should have a bundle of straw hung outside it for forty days, on a pole at least ten feet long overhanging the street, and that everyone from an infected household was to carry a white rod four feet long whenever they went out. In addition to these requirements, a plague victim's clothes were not to be worn for three months after their death. The distinguishing marker on an infected house proved to be too elaborate, and in September 1521 the bundle of straw was replaced by a headless cross, known as a St Anthony's Cross, fixed on the front of the building.

The regulations were designed to clearly identify infected houses and individuals and so to isolate the sick, and reflected the view that the disease was contagious. They also acknowledged that the government had a role in public health matters, and were among a number of interventionist policies which Wolsey initiated in the years after he came to power. These included an enquiry into enclosures, sumptuary laws which sought to regulate 'excessive fare' by setting the appropriate numbers of courses for meals, specified by social rank from cardinals downwards, and, in London, a campaign against beggars, vagrants and prostitutes, the fixing of the price of poultry and an investigation into the reasons for the scarcity of meat. There was also an order for the cleaning of the streets, 'for the avoiding of contagious infections'.

Another development during the period, while attention was focused on public health, was the establishment in 1518 of the Royal College of Physicians of London. This was set up by royal charter, under the influence of Thomas Linacre, with powers to license and oversee medical practice, and to punish unlicensed practitioners and prevent them from practising. Originally consisting of twenty fellows, the College's functions included providing advice and information respecting plague in London. But treatment of epidemic disease was not generally regarded as one of the physicians' functions. According to Thomas Starkey, writing between 1529 and 1532, they had become necessary in cities and towns because 'men commynly gyve themselfe to such inordynat dyat', and less gluttony and more self-restraint would make them unnecessary. Diet was associated with disease, including plague. In 1528 Anne Boleyn, who was being courted assiduously by the king, wrote to Wolsey that she was pleased to hear that he had escaped the plague and hoped that it was declining, 'especially with those who keep good diet, as I trust you do'.

The procedure for implementing the health and environmental regulations, followed in 1518 and subsequently, was for the Privy Council to recommend measures to the Lord Mayor and aldermen, who issued precepts requiring the measures to be carried out by the ward and parish officers. But if the regulations of January 1518 were designed partly to allay the king's anxious fear of plague, then they failed. His apprehension returned with warm weather in April and he again withdrew, to the Abingdon area, explaining to the Council that he could not come to London because of the danger of the plague, a decision reinforced by the queen's gloomy prediction that something 'inconvenient' would befall the king's person if he returned. He spent the spring and summer moving around, first in the Thames valley and then, driven away from there by the plague, in Hertfordshire, afraid to return to London while the disease raged there. Part of the problem was that the royal accommodation at Westminster Palace had been destroyed by fire in 1512 and not rebuilt, and Bridewell was being converted as the new royal residence in the capital. Close to the confluence of the Thames and the Fleet, this was much more central than Westminster and in a densely populated part of the city, with implications for the court's exposure to disease.

The government required more information if it was to assess the extent of the risk, and whether the number of plague cases was increasing or declining. In 1519 the Lord Mayor was directed to compile the necessary statistics, a task which should have been made easier by the isolation of the plague victims and their houses required in the proclamation of the previous year. The survey was carried out, and at the end of August a return was made to Wolsey of the numbers who had died of the 'common sickness' since the beginning of the enquiry.

Cities in north-west Europe had previously introduced measures which anticipated the London regulations and may have served as models. At Lille, in 1480, plague victims were required to carry a rod three feet long while they were in public places, and orders for marking infected houses had been introduced in Paris in 1510. Regulations issued in Edinburgh in 1505 and amplified in 1512 required cases of sickness to be reported within twenty-four hours and ordered that those with plague should not leave their houses without the pest-officers' approval, and then only if they carried a white rod or wore a white cross on their chest. Provision was also made for the detection of infected houses, the restriction of movement of the sick and the culling of stray dogs, cats and pigs.

The regulations first introduced in London in 1518–19 were gradually developed over the following decades, as plague

returned intermittently. It continued to worry the king, especially in 1525: 'In this Wynter was greate death in London,
wherefore the Terme was adjorned, and the king for to eschew
the plague, kept his Christmas at Eltham with a small nomber,
for no manne might come thether, but such as wer appoynted
by name.' An outbreak in the following year was probably
responsible for the death of the Venetian ambassador, and there
was an epidemic of the sweat in 1525–26. This was now less
deadly than when it first reached England. In 1528 the king
told Anne Boleyn of five members of the household, including
the apothecary, who had contracted the disease and recovered,
and in the following year both Anne and Cardinal Wolsey contracted it and survived. Even so, it still engendered great alarm,
to the extent that one observer thought that some succumbed
to the symptoms without being sick, purely through fear, which
was spread and intensified by gossip. The king continued to
take evasive action, recommended others to keep 'out of all air
where any of that infection is' and expressed his opinions on
the suitable treatment for victims. His nervous anxiety, and the
fear of contagion, prompted those who prepared accusations
of misconduct against the cardinal after his fall from power
to allege that he had contracted syphilis, yet 'endangered the
king's person in that he, when he knew himself to have the
foul and contagious disease of the great pox broken out upon
him in divers places of his body, came daily to your grace,
rowning [speaking] in your ear and blowing upon your most
noble grace with his perilous and infective breath'.

The sweat and other diseases did not deflect attention from
plague, which was dangerous enough in 1528 for figures to be
compiled of the number of plague deaths and the parishes which
were free from the disease. Similar returns were prepared in 1532,
on the orders of the Privy Council to the Lord Mayor, in a year
when plague was reported to be widespread in London, with
the area around Fleet Street and the Temple especially badly

affected. In late October, three-quarters of the 126 recorded
deaths were attributed to plague. The records for 1535 show
that over a four-week period during the warm and wet summer
there were 303 deaths from plague, which was said to be present
in every London parish, although the Lord Mayor defiantly
asserted that the extent of the disease was exaggerated and so he
would not cancel St Bartholomew's Fair. Prohibition of the fair
and visits by Londoners to fairs elsewhere, cancellation of the
Law term (with the courts meeting elsewhere), the proroguing
of Parliament and proclamations forbidding anyone going from
London to court became common measures during epidemics.
All were economically harmful to the city, and sources of tension between the Privy Council and the corporation.

The recording of the numbers of plague deaths should have
removed much of the uncertainty regarding the incidence of
plague, with facts replacing speculation. But the figures were
open to interpretation, influenced by economic self-interest
as well as fear. In July 1537 the Archbishop of Canterbury,
Thomas Cranmer, asked for permission to leave London
because of the mortality across the city, yet on the very same
day the weekly number of plague deaths was cited to show
that the disease was not as serious as in the previous year. Such
apparently contradictory responses did not diminish the value
of the returns, which evolved into the Bills of Mortality, an
increasingly informative set of figures on the numbers, causes
and locations of deaths. Intended to provide the authorities
with data about the prevalence and distribution of the disease,
they were also consulted by those anxious not to delay their
departure from the city as an epidemic developed. Record-
keeping was extended in 1538 when Thomas Cromwell, as
Vicar General, ordered that a record be kept of the baptisms,
marriages and burials in every parish, and some clerks chose
to note the cause of death, especially plague, in their parish
register. In 1555 this became a requirement, when they were

directed to make returns of the numbers 'of all the persons that do die and whereof they die'.

The increasing availability of statistics did nothing to diminish royal anxiety during the 1530s. Following Wolsey's fall from favour and his death, the king appropriated York Place, which, as Whitehall Palace, became the principal royal palace in London until it was destroyed by fire in 1698. Further away from the densely populated parts of the capital than Bridewell, it should have been a safer place, although not entirely secure from infection. Enlargement of the site included the incorporation of the road used for taking to burial the corpses of parishioners of St Margaret's who had died in St Martin's. This prompted a letter from the king to the abbot of Westminster in 1535, a year in which 'the contagious plague called the Great Sickness' in and around London caused the prorogation of Parliament. He directed that all those living in St Martin's should be treated as if they were its parishioners, ending the practice of moving infected bodies and the consequent danger posed by the 'goeing & comeing by the Infect Persons accompying the Dead Persons & Bodys as by the Infection of their Cloaths & otherwise'. In 1542, this was formalised by the annexation of that part of St Margaret's north of Whitehall to St Martin's. Among other steps taken to protect the royal family was control of those allowed to attend the baptism in October 1537 of Prince Edward, the king's longed-for male heir, because of the 'great infection of the plague' in London.

The wisdom of avoiding crowds and keeping company only with those known to be free from infection was becoming widely accepted and was endorsed by contemporary writers. One of the works translated into English by Thomas Paynel, canon of Merton Abbey and later a chaplain to the king, was published in 1534 as *A moche profitable treatise against the pestilence*. It included the shrewd advice that 'greate multitude and congregation of people' should be avoided, because 'in a greatte multytude maye be some one infectyd the which may infecte manye'. Thomas Phayre, in 1545, was sure that 'venomous air' was nowhere near as dangerous as the conversation or breath of those who were infected already, although his comment may have had a moral as well as a medical purpose, equating the discourse of heretic Lutherans with pestilence. Careful behaviour by individuals, coupled with a sense of social responsibility, could provide some degree of security during plague outbreaks. Carelessness or selfishness, on the other hand, were condemned. In 1541, the servant of one of the members of the Inner Temple died in his chamber during 'the sickness', without any warning or information being given to the others, and when this was discovered the house had to disperse and the member was reprimanded and fined.

As well as judicious behaviour by individuals, the corporation was expected to fulfil its duties by enforcing regulations and overseeing good practices by the wards and parishes. A plague epidemic in 1543 prompted the Privy Council to reprimand the Lord Mayor for negligence in a number of respects, and they sent him instructions, which were then issued to the wards. Infected houses should be distinctly marked with a cross, which was to remain for forty days, and the sick who could live on their own resources were not to go out and into others' company for a month. But the Council recognised that the poor did need to obtain money and provisions, and ruled that they should be allowed in public places if they carried a white rod, two feet long, for forty days after the symptoms had appeared. No householder was to expel a sick person unless other accommodation had been found first; in other words, turning someone out of a house into the street to become a beggar because they had the plague was not permitted.

Beggars were tolerated, but regarded as health risks, and in 1538 the 'myserable people lyeng in the streete' had been described as 'offendyng every clene person passyng by the waye

with theyre fylthye and nastye savors'. Churchwardens were
now ordered to keep them out of the churches during services,
to safeguard the parishioners' health. Dogs were to be taken
from the city or killed, except for hounds, spaniels and mastiffs
kept as guard dogs. Straw and rushes had to be carried out of the
city, and the clothes of plague victims aired in the fields, and not
hung outside houses or from windows. Most of the measures
dealt with the potential threat from contagion, although the
danger from miasmic air was recognised in the orders that the
water should be drawn from the wells and the streets and alleys
should be kept clean. Harsh penalties were stipulated for those
breaking any of the regulations, with imprisonment for twenty
days and expulsion from the freedom of the City, which had
serious implications for earning a living. In early October, the
Privy Council also reminded the Lord Mayor that he should
be sending weekly returns of the numbers of plague deaths. He
replied that he had been compiling the returns since 27 April,
and countered the complaint by pointing out that he needed
to be provided with a designated messenger or given a place
where the returns could be deposited for collection, for all of
his own officers had been required to go into infected areas
and so would break the order given in the royal proclamation
if they went to court with the figures.

The epidemic in London in 1543 was a serious one,
beginning in the spring and still so bad in October, when the
city was described as 'sore infected with the pestilence', that the
law courts met in St Albans. In eighteen parishes the number
of burials was roughly twice the average for the decade, and
eighteen plague burials were recorded in the small parish of
St Pancras, Soper Lane, on the south side of Poultry, a higher
number than in any other year between 1538 and 1599.

Henry VIII died in January 1547 and was succeeded by
his son Edward. This did not mark any change in policy
regarding access to the court during plague outbreaks. In both

1544 and 1547 epidemics prompted royal proclamations, forbidding anyone who lived in a house where someone had fallen
ill with the plague, had visited a house containing a plague
victim, or lived near an infected house, from going to court,
and forbidding anyone from the court to enter those houses.
In 1547, the order to display a St Anthony's cross on a house
where an infected person had lived was repeated; the cross was
painted blue. A more serious epidemic in 1548 caused a 'great
mortalitie' in London, with the number of plague victims in the
sample of eighteen parishes as high as in 1543, although four
fewer plague victims were buried at St Pancras. In St Lawrence
Jewry, another central parish, burials were more than six times
the normal level in 1548 and slightly more than in 1543.

Funeral practices during epidemics had attracted attention
already, as the authorities attempted to prevent parishioners
from observing the usual rituals. An injunction by the bishop
of London, Edmund Bonner, in 1542 had directed that during
plagues bodies were not to be taken into the churches, but
straight to the graves and buried immediately, 'whereby the
people may the rather avoid infection'. The hours of burial
were regulated by an order issued in 1548, with the clergy
instructed not to conduct burials before six o'clock in the
morning or after six in the evening, coupled with the instruction that for each interment one bell should be rung for at least
three-quarters of an hour. The frequent tolling of the passing
bell was a characteristic and depressing feature of epidemics
and the purpose of this order may have been to ensure that
the practice was properly observed, perhaps to emphasise the
severity of the outbreak and so induce more care in implementing the regulations.

The plague year of 1548 was followed by three successive poor harvests and so rising food prices, ushering in the
bad decade of the 1550s. To make matters worse, in 1550
and 1551 the London Merchant Adventurers encountered

serious problems marketing their cloth at Antwerp, by far their largest and most profitable outlet, due to an unfavourable exchange rate and a campaign by Charles V against heretics in the Low Countries. In 1551 the sweat returned with a short but sharp epidemic in which 'there dyde a grett multitude of pepull sodenly thorrow alle London'. Within the space of three weeks in July, between 1,000 and 1,100 people died of the disease, generally within twenty-four hours. The scale of the death toll was blamed on the lack of guidance for treating the sick. Although the outbreak was relatively short, the nature of the illness, the speed of death and the deaths of those who had seemed to be 'in best health' made such an impact that the epidemic was remembered as 'a terrible time in London'. The decade also saw outbreaks of plague; in 1554 a visitor noted that, 'They have some little plague in England every year, for which they are not accustomed to make sanitary provisions.' The situation was not altered by changes of monarch during the 1550s. Edward VI died in July 1553 and was succeeded by his elder sister, Mary, whose reign lasted just over five years until her death in November 1558, a period which was marked by economic and demographic problems. On her death her sister Elizabeth, who had no heir, came to the throne.

The bad harvest of 1555 was followed in 1556 by the worst harvest of the century and in 1557–59 by an influenza epidemic across the country. The outbreak was so destructive that the late 1550s was probably the only period between 1540 and the 1650s when the increase in England's population was checked and there was a decline. In 1558–59 the mortality rate was more than twice the long-term average, and at least 8,000 people died in London during the epidemic. A rise in the enrolments of apprentices over the next three years indicates a recovery of the capital's population, but this was halted in 1563 by a terrible outbreak of plague.

Le Havre had been occupied in the previous October by an English force in support of the Huguenot armies. The garrison was besieged in May 1563 and at the beginning of June plague appeared within the town. It spread rapidly, producing a death toll of sixty a day by the end of the month and double that number at the end of July, with a total of 2,600 deaths by the time that the garrison surrendered, just over a third of the men deployed in the operation. The danger that the returning soldiers could spread the disease was recognised by the government, which ordered that they should keep their contacts with others to a minimum and that the authorities in places where the soldiers arrived should designate sites where they could be isolated and supplied with provisions. These measures were probably impractical and unenforceable, but demonstrate that the government believed that isolation could control the spread of epidemic disease.

The orders were issued too late to prevent an outbreak in London, which, according to the College of Physicians, began on 1 June in Shoe Lane, Holborn, spreading first in the area around Long Lane, off Smithfield, and then across the city. The date suggests that the infection did not necessarily come from the garrison of Le Havre. July saw a rising death toll from plague, with 289 burials in the City and thirty-one in the out parishes in the last week of the month. This was a high enough number to cause the queen to leave for Windsor. With the dynasty again as fragile as in the early years of Henry VIII's reign, gallows were erected in the marketplace as a deterrent to anyone from London who might have been tempted to enter the town. Those who were due to make payment into the government's coffers were instructed to do so at Syon House, near Brentford.

Existing arrangements for collecting statistics during epidemics were implemented and maintained. The returns show that the numbers of plague deaths more than trebled during

August, from 299 in the first week to 976 three weeks later, continuing to rise during the early autumn, to peak at 1,828 deaths in the week ending 1 October. They remained high until the end of that month, when the corporation believed that the plague 'dothe more and more encrese', and did not fall below 100 per week until January 1564. Indeed, the number of deaths attributed to plague in December was thirty-one per cent higher than in July.

The total number of deaths in the City and surrounding parishes during the year was 23,660, of which 20,136, or eighty-five per cent, were attributed to plague, with an overall mortality rate of roughly twenty per cent of the total population. The number of burials within the City was 7.7 times the pre-plague level, and in some parishes was even higher. Burials recorded at St Mary Aldermary and St Dionis Backchurch were 8.5 times the level of the preceding years, with October the peak month in both parishes, and in St Thomas the Apostle was almost twelve times higher. Theirs were typical experiences in the central districts, for the ten parishes with the highest recorded mortality during the outbreak all lay within the city walls.

The mounting death toll produced the common dilemma, whether or not to flee. This was eloquently expressed by characters in William Bullein's *A Dialogue against the Pestilence*, published in the following year. A citizen grows fearful because of the unmistakable indications of an unfolding epidemic: 'the daily jangling and ringing of the bells, the coming in of the Minister to every house in ministring the communion, in reading the homily of death, the digging up of graves, the sparring in of windows, and the blazing forth of the blue cross'. He has not had direct experience of plague or death, yet what he sees and hears makes him so fearful for his own safety that he asks his wife 'what shall I do to save my life?'. Hers is the voice of reason, as she replies that they are still young, asks why they should stay to accumulate money if they will not live to enjoy it, and points out that they have already sent their children to the country three weeks earlier 'into a good air'. They should now follow them, say goodbye to their neighbours and return only 'when the plague is past, and the dog days ended'.

By mid-September, 'a greate number' of the aldermen had come to that conclusion and left. John Stow recalled that 'the rich by flight into the countries made shift for themselves', while the poor who remained suffered not only from the plague, but also because of a shortage of money and scarcity of provisions, 'the miserie whereof were too long here to write'. Among those who did not leave were the members of Mr Revelle's household in St Dionis parish, where one child, two apprentices and three servants died, and the family of Gregory Yong, in St Peter's, Cornhill, whose wife was buried on 10 September and his daughter two days later. The compilation of the Bills of Mortality throughout the epidemic indicates that parish officers remained and fulfilled their duties. At St Michael's, Cornhill they paid for the construction of pest-houses to isolate the sick. John Webb, alias Clarke, the parish clerk of St Dionis, had lived through many sickly years by the time that he died in February 1564. He came to the parish in 1516: 'And hys sarvys so dylygent to ye p'ishe, that he never lay nyght owt of the same p'ishe all the same tyme, but allwayes watyng on hys sarvyse.'

The Dutch community, of about 1,600 people, appointed a surgeon and arranged for visitors of the sick and the issue of health certificates for those who had recovered from the disease. The ministers remained at their posts, comforting the sick, and the two most senior ones died in September, within a few days of each other. Peter Docket, a physician in St Mary Aldermary, and his family also stayed, and between 29 October and 13 December three of his sons and three daughters died. But despite such devotion to duty, physicians were blamed for not healing as many as they were expected to do, and some

patients would not take their advice, but listened instead to
self-appointed experts without qualifications holding forth at
'the ale bench and gosseping cup'. John Jones, a physician,
complained that they misled others by claiming that someone
who had survived an attack of plague was then immune. To
contradict this, he cited the case of a woman who lived beyond
Temple Bar who twice survived bouts of the disease in 1563,
but died of a third attack later in the year.

Implementation of the orders issued by the Lord Mayor was
also uneven during such a crisis, not helped by the absence
of some aldermen. Yet the corporation acted quickly and on
3 July issued orders for the fixing of 'blew hedles Crosses' on
infected houses, the flushing of gutters to clean them and the
burning of bedding. It ordered 400 crosses, which had been
distributed by the middle of the month, when an instruction
was issued that they should be set up on houses in which
anyone had been infected within the previous six days. The
parish clerks were to check every morning that none had been
taken down and to replace those which had been removed.
Household quarantine was to be enforced, with those in an
infected house remaining there for a month, although one
person was permitted to go out for provisions if carrying a
white rod two feet long. Both miasmic and contagious risks
were addressed, with the direction that fires should be lit in
the streets on three evenings each week, to circulate stagnant
air, and the observation that dogs going around the city and
from house to house were spreading the plague by carrying
with them corrupt air and infection. They could now be taken
out only if on a lead, and strays were to be killed by the dog-
catcher. The corporation seems to have regarded the outbreak
as an opportunity to deal with other problems caused by dogs,
for the barking of 'the great multitude of dogges' disturbed the
citizens during the nights, when they should be getting their
rest, and were also the cause of quarrels and disturbances.

In August, fines were specified for those breaking the regulations, and for the clerks, constables and churchwardens who were not enforcing them. Half of the sums collected were to go to the poor, but in early September the spectacle of beggars with the plague lying in the streets prompted an order that all parishes should also take a special collection for the poor, as some already had done. Recognising that the wealthier citizens might have gone, the proclamation ordered that information about the collection should be left with the servants and housekeepers in those houses, presumably hoping that they could pass the news on and then be told to contribute to it. But the fundraising was not as successful as had been hoped and the aldermen were instructed to summon the vicars and churchwardens once a week, to ensure that the sums collected were being distributed.

Landlords were ordered not to take tenants into houses or rooms that were empty because their occupants had died of plague, and the constables were told to search the alleys and lanes and send lists of such houses to the Lord Mayor. No householder was to take in anyone who had not been living in London for the previous three months. This must have been difficult to enforce and, although breach of the order carried a penalty of six months' imprisonment, in November it had to be admitted that many poor people were coming to London and moving into accommodation where infected people had lived.

The effect of such an epidemic in London was an economic downturn in the surrounding areas, creating a pool of people who had little to lose by moving to the city itself in search of a living. They hoped to be able to take advantage of the opportunities left by those who had died or fled, and the risk of catching plague was outweighed by the likelihood of finding work or another worthwhile opening, and free lodging in empty houses. Nor could they be sure of safety from plague if they remained outside London, as the disease spread. But their recklessness was clearly alarming, for they came 'hoping of gayne and lucre and very litle or nothing at all fearing the great plague'. This was happening on such a scale as to attract the attention of the corporation and, as the epidemic began to wane, in December a search of inns, other hostelries and victualling houses was ordered, for idle persons, vagabonds and 'masterless men'.

The aim of preventing the spread of the disease by restricting contact with people who might be contagious was, in any case, confused by the Lord Mayor's own order in mid-August regarding worship. This required that the clergy should hold services at eight o'clock every morning and that at least one person from every house, and preferably two, should attend and remain for at least an hour. Tavern-keepers and victuallers were not to serve customers during the hours of service on Wednesdays and Fridays, nor should anyone play sports at those times. To reduce the risk of the disease spreading, the church-wardens were to sweep and clean the churches and to remove some of the glass from the windows to let in clean air.

The policy echoed that of the bishop of London, Edmund Grindal, who issued a form of worship for use during the epidemic and directed the clergy to exhort their parishioners 'diligently to frequent the common prayer' in their parish churches. Gatherings in the larger churches, such as Christ Church, Newgate Street, were not favoured, however, because such meetings 'might be occasion to spread the infection'. Church congregations were not regarded in the same way as audiences watching plays and interludes. In February 1564, such entertainments were prohibited unless licensed by the Lord Mayor. They were performed at inns and the ban was justified on the grounds that people assembling and crowding together risked the spread of the plague. This restriction had not been introduced earlier, while the plague was far more extensive, and yet it related morality with health, public performances being associated with sinfulness and so liable to provoke the wrath of God, through plague. Grindal asked for a ban for a year on plays within three miles of the city, with the comment that 'if it were for ever it would not be amiss'.

The epidemic continued into 1564, and the removal of the court and the holding of the Law term at Hertford caused 'greate decay, losse and hinderance' to innkeepers and victuallers in London, as well as to 'many artificers and handy craftsmen'. The economic consequences of the outbreak were exacerbated by the decision of Margaret, Duchess of Parma, Philip II's half-sister and regent in the Netherlands, to prohibit trade with London because of the plague. Exports to London were stopped and so were imports, which seriously affected the cloth trade with Antwerp. The London merchants negotiated an alternative outlet at Emden. Although that arrangement was short-lived, a longer breach of trade with Antwerp began in 1568, with the outbreak of the Dutch revolt.

Quarantining of the sick as soon as possible remained a principal objective of the policy for containing plague, with other orders issued according to circumstances and perceived risks to health. An abundant fruit harvest in 1569 prompted a warning about the sale of fruit in the streets, presumably because it could rot and corrupt the air. John Jones thought that the most polluted places in the city were in St Sepulchre's parish, because of its 'many fruterers, pore people, and stinking lanes'. The practice of the pudding and tripe cooks of emptying their tubs and pails into the streets, rather than the Thames, was also condemned. Searches for beggars were conducted occasionally, although they were not always harshly dealt with. In 1569, the Lord Mayor ordered that the homeless lying in the fields or 'under stalles or at menns dores' were to be taken to St Thomas' and St Bartholomew's hospitals, which were directed to admit them.

The period of quarantine was reduced to twenty days in 1570, and this was maintained for the next few years. The longer periods of four weeks or forty days were expensive in terms of providing for those quarantined, and less likely to be willingly observed. In 1574, orders were issued that the words 'The Lord have mercy upon us' should be fixed to infected houses, and that two people should be appointed in each parish to examine the body of anyone suspected to have died of plague, to decide if it had been the cause of death. Two more women were to take provisions to those who were being held in quarantine, making it unnecessary for anyone from those houses to go out. The parishes seem to have complied with the requirements. St Margaret's Lothbury appointed two women searchers in September 1574 to scrutinise suspect bodies, at 3d per examination. In 1573 St Christopher-le-Stocks bought 'red wandes and bylles for the plague' and in 1582–83 St Michael's, Cornhill and St Botolph's-without-Aldersgate also purchased rods for the sick to carry when they went out. Red had replaced white as the specified colour, and the policy of keeping everyone within an infected house evidently was not entirely effective, or they would not have been needed. A baker's wife, in 1570, cared for a friend who had the plague, going to her almost daily, regardless of the quarantine regulations, and spending five or six hours at her bedside on the night before she died.

The problems of enforcement were well known and in 1577 the Privy Council sent an enquiry under six headings asking for information on breaches of the orders. One problem was that parish officers concealed information of plague cases or did not execute the orders, 'either for corruption or friendship', so that the healthy unwittingly mixed with plague victims in the streets and at the shops. Another was social partiality: 'either in restraining the poor upon infection of plague more than the rich, or in sparing the rich transgressing the good orders taken for the stay of the infection, and punishing the poorer sort'. A distinction certainly existed in burial practice during epidemics, with funerals prohibited during divine service, 'excepte it be some personn of honor or Worshipp'.

The Council's doubts regarding the concealment of the numbers of plague victims arose again in 1578. The weekly returns were being made, but it thought that the number of cases was being understated 'by the corruption and indirect dealing of some inferior minister', and William Cecil, Lord Burghley complained to the Lord Mayor of his neglect in not enforcing the regulations. In his response, the mayor pointed to the scale of the problem in such a populous city, and the failings of the citizens, 'either in the inferior officers who seek not so carefully to discharge their duty, or in the people, who will hardly conceive what is for their good provided'. Of course, fear for personal safety hindered the implementation of the City's policies. The local officers were afraid to pursue their enquiries too far in the areas where plague was present and the inhabitants were antagonistic, and if they were persistent and contracted the disease they might pass it on to their superiors. Nevertheless, some of the senior officials conscientiously made inspections. Sir William Fleetwood, the City's Recorder, had attended to his duties, having people with plague sores coming to him daily, and going around the city looking for beggars, until the shock of finding corpses under tables in the houses he entered became too much and he retreated to Buckinghamshire for a respite. Burghley's concern was no doubt aroused by the level of plague deaths that year, with 3,500 deaths from plague within the City and liberties and 2.3 times the average number of burials.

During the epidemic of 1563, Cesare Aldemare, an Italian physician in London, had suggested to Burghley that measures such as those taken by the Italian cities should be adopted. Nothing had been done at the time, but following the severe

plague epidemic in Italy in 1576 – causing mortality rates
of twenty-eight per cent in Venice and eighteen per cent
in Milan – the Privy Council acquired copies of the orders
issued in Milan during the crisis. Closer to home, plague
was spreading through the Low Countries in 1577. A draft
set of regulations to be executed 'throughout the realm' was
prepared early in 1578 and revised later in the year, after the
College of Physicians had been consulted, and was then issued
as a printed set of orders. London was exempt, after a consultation. In November, the Privy Council ordered the Lord
Mayor to send to a meeting the Recorder and two aldermen
who lived as far as possible from areas infected by plague, and
soon afterwards provided a draft of twenty-two articles for
the City's consideration. They included proposals for weekly
taxation, the compilation of lists of inhabitants, which were to
be checked weekly to avoid secret burials, a listing of houses
in multiple occupancy, and the appointment of overseers and
paid physicians, apothecaries and clergymen, who were to
care for the sick.

The City prevaricated and made clear its preference for the
existing system of aldermen and parish officers rather than paid
officials, and voluntary contributions rather than a weekly tax,
and pointed out that a census of houses and inhabitants would
be difficult to administer. The arrangements which resulted
from the consultation retained the structure of aldermen, ward
and parish officials, but they were to be assisted by two general
overseers appointed monthly in each ward by the aldermen.
Parish collections were to be taken weekly and physicians and
apothecaries paid for attending the poor, not given an annual
stipend. The Lord Mayor warned the aldermen to go through
their wards once a week, to ensure that the overseers were
executing the precepts and punishing the defaulters 'without
respect of persons'. Yet the City did ask for help in the establishment of a hospital or pesthouse, 'where maye be certen

officers and orders as in other countries'. Isolation hospitals
had been set up in a number of continental cities from the early
fifteenth century, the best known and most widely admired
of which was Milan's Lazaretto di San Gregorio, built in 1488.
More recently, the Dutch city of Utrecht had erected a pesthouse in 1567. Nothing was done to provide a similar building
for London before 1594, although some individual parishes
had made such provision for their own plague victims.

Another development, of long-term significance and perhaps suggested by continental practice, was the authorisation
by the Privy Council in June 1580, at the Lord Mayor's own
suggestion, for the detaining of ships from Lisbon (which was
in the grip of a plague epidemic), Plymouth, or anywhere
else suffering from the disease. Their cargoes could not be
unloaded before they had been aired, or their crews and
passengers disembarked until they had served a period of quarantine. This followed attempts by the Privy Council in 1579 to
prevent carriers from Norwich, Salisbury and Great Yarmouth,
where the plague was present, from coming to Bartholomew's
Fair, with an order that the Great Yarmouth fishermen should
not bring their herrings to London. In 1585 similar orders
were issued, with traffic from Bordeaux and other ports on
the River Garonne banned because of plague there, anyone
from Norwich or other places suffering the plague prohibited
from coming to London, and Londoners forbidden to receive
goods or visitors from those places.

Such steps to restrict both internal and overseas trade with
infected places were not included in the printed orders for
London. These were issued in May 1583, under twenty-one
heads, and codified existing practices. Household quarantine
was retained, including anyone who entered an infected house,
with the period of closure now set at twenty-eight days. Two
women were appointed in each parish to supply the closed
houses with provisions, yet one person was to be allowed out

for the same purpose, carrying a red rod three feet long and avoiding others as they went along the streets. Even more surprisingly, those in an infected house could leave the city, but not return within twenty-eight days, which would reduce the burden of providing for the closed houses by shifting the problem to the surrounding areas.

The sealing off of a neighbourhood with plague had been tried at Leicester and Gloucester, and at Venice during the outbreak in 1576, when no one was allowed to move between streets for a fourteen-day period, but the strategy evidently was not favoured in London. It would have been an expensive policy to implement, with provision having to be made for so many houses, including those of the healthy as well as the sick. The corporation wanted to target assistance to those genuinely in need, not extend it to those able to provide for themselves. And plague increasingly was becoming associated with the housing of the poor in the alleys and back lanes, and not that of the more affluent citizens fronting the principal streets. The better-off families would have greatly resented being confined to their houses.

The Italian model of a board of health with overall authority was not adopted, although there was a clear structure for super-vision, with the alderman of each ward and his deputy, and the two surveyors of each parish, responsible for seeing that the orders were observed. Among the junior officers, the scaven-gers and rakers were to ensure that the streets were cleaned and properly paved, so that there was no cavity where rubbish might collect and putrefy, and the 'sober anciente women' appointed as searchers of the bodies were to be imprisoned if they neglected their duty, and to stand in the pillory if they made false returns of the cause of death. Physicians and sur-geons were to treat only plague victims during the epidemic and were to be paid for attending to poor patients; those who could pay were to meet the costs of their treatment. Other clauses repeated previous orders, with rules for burials, the disposal or cleansing of clothing and bedding, the killing of dogs who strayed, or howled and annoyed the neighbours, and a ban on plays and interludes. Displaying these printed orders around the city was aimed at helping the officers to get compliance from the citizens.

An underlying concern was the numbers of poor and homeless and the cost of assisting them. Accommodation was becoming overcrowded, reflecting the rapid growth of the city, leading to insanitary conditions and unpleasant smells, reinforcing the belief that 'yll savors in the streets is one of the greatest occasions of the infection of plague'. The increasing number of strangers, defined as 'suche as be of no churche', was one of the points made in response to the Privy Council's draft regulations in 1578. The foreigners were culpable because they received 'infected stuffe out of the lowe countries' and were a cause of poverty among native workers. If they could be found and removed, overcrowding would be reduced. Such anxiety led to investigations of the numbers. In 1562, fewer than 5,000 foreign immigrants were discovered in the capital and in 1573 there were 7,143, roughly a third of whom admitted coming primarily for economic reasons.

Although the number of strangers was relatively small, there was visible evidence of overcrowding and, increasingly, environmental conditions and public health were linked together in the policies pursued by the Privy Council and the corporation. The population of London rose remorselessly, from perhaps 75,000 in 1550 to 200,000 in 1600, and came to be a major concern to Elizabeth's government, so much so that in 1580 a proclamation was issued prohibiting new building and pronouncing that every house should be occupied by only one family. The poor living conditions were seen as a threat to health, for:

...where there are such great multitudes of people brought to inhabit in small rooms, whereof a great part are seen very poor, yea, such as must live of begging, or by worse means, and they heaped up together, and in a sort smothered with many families of children and servants in one house or small tenement; it must needs follow, if any plague or popular sickness should, by God's permission, enter amongst those multitudes, that the same would not only spread itself, and invade the whole city and confines, but that a great mortality would ensue...

Because of the numbers coming to London, to the courts or on business, there would also be a danger that the disease could be spread through the country when they returned home.

According to John Howes, of the Grocers' Company, a great deal of money was paid in poor relief and St Bartholomew's and St Thomas' hospitals together treated roughly 850 people each year, at a cost of £1,600, without any visible effect. Londoners were too busy with their own affairs to be able to watch the streets for beggars, and the parish beadles were afraid of contact with them in case they carried the plague. As a result:

...the streates yet swarme with beggers, that no man can stande or staie in any churche or streate, but presently tenne or twelve beggers comme breathing in his face, many of them having theire plague sores and other contageous disseases running on them, wandring from man to man to seke relefe, which is very daungerous to all hir maiesties good subiects, and the very highe waie to infect the whole kingdomme.

He was writing in 1587 and commented on the 'great nomber of poore men, which have died this sommer of the sycknes in the streats for want of reliefe'. The many beggars and poor in London included soldiers who were wounded or look-ing for employment, as the city was the principal place for recruitment; men and women in service seeking a new post after they had been dismissed or their master had died; aimless young men who spent freely and so were gaoled for debt or a violent affray; and children from the country who wandered the streets, either because work was irregular and when it was scarce they were laid off, or because they were treated so harshly that they ran away. The overcrowding which resulted was exploited by the landlords of properties in the alleys, who charged high rents and compelled their tenants to buy their provisions through them. Local bakers, brewers, victuallers and maltsters benefited from such arrangements, which gave them a captive market, and so were unwilling to tackle the problem while they were serving as parish officers. The cottages were so dirty they were not fit for dogs to live in, and were over-crowded, with three or four tenants living in a room without a chimney or privy.

Howes drew a grim picture of the conditions for the poor in Elizabethan London, but also suggested measures which would ameliorate them. The aldermen and churchwardens could oversee the numbers of tenants in a property, and a minimum age of eighteen could be enforced to prevent young children coming to London. But his proposals to remove the 'lowsie and fylthie cottages' were the most radical, with the recommendation that the corporation, its Bridgehouse com-mittee or the livery companies could buy the properties in the alleys and demolish them, replacing them with convenient lodgings at reasonable rents, acting as model landlords. He had in mind the Fuggerei, a housing development built for the poor of Augsburg by Jakob Fugger. Begun in 1514, the district contained small houses, each of three rooms, in eight streets, with its own church and enclosing wall. Such slum clearance and rebuilding would remove the unhealthy places where the landlords housed too many tenants without providing privies. But neither the finances nor the administrative organisation were available to implement such a programme, even if the political will had been there, and a proposal for the City to purchase all of the properties within the area destroyed in the Great Fire in 1666 was to be stillborn for similar reasons. Yet Howes' scheme, and the government's growing concern with housing, show an awareness that the impact of plague could be reduced by improving living conditions.

The printed plague orders and Howes' proposals came towards the end of a period during which plague had struck fairly frequently. The Michaelmas Law term was adjourned from Westminster in every year between 1574 and 1582, with the sole exception of 1580. Even in 1580 there were 128 plague deaths, with probably more than 1,000 in 1581, and in 1582 plague caused 2,976 of the 6,762 recorded deaths. Plays and other public entertainments again attracted attention, both for the risk of the infection being spread in crowds, which included 'the basest sort of people' and those who already had the plague, and their corrupting influence. In 1574, Thomas Norton's advice 'towchinge the contagion of sickenes' included avoiding the 'unnecessarie and scarslie honest resorts to plaies, to shewes to thoccasion of thronges and presse, except to the servyce of God; and especiallie the assemblies to the unchaste, shamelesse and unnaturall tomblinge of the Italian Weomen'. He made the distinction between crowds assembled for worship and those who gathered at entertainments, with a topical condemnation of the performances by women acrobats.

When preaching a sermon at Paul's Cross in November 1577, 'in the time of the plague', Thomas White, vicar of St Dunstan's-in-the-West, made the deduction that plays were the cause of sin. Commenting that he supported the policy of forbidding plays during the plague, he added that 'a disease is but bodged or patched up that is not cured in the cause, and the cause of plagues is sinne, if you looke to it well: and the cause of sinne are playes: therefore the cause of plagues are playes'. He may have been provoked by a recent development, the building of playhouses. London's first, the Theatre, had been opened in Shoreditch in the previous year, and 1577 saw the building of a second, the Curtain, in the same district. Many others condemned plays, for drawing the citizens away from their work and creating disturbances, and as fundamentally immoral. The City authorities saw them as 'ungodlye and perilous' and not only supported the Council's orders to ban performances during plagues, but on occasion suggested that action. Closure of the playhouses became a characteristic of plague epidemics, together with reiteration of the orders to protect the court, adjourn the Law term and slaughter domestic animals.

Mortality levels in 1582 were high enough to draw attention to the problem of burials. Population growth had produced pressure on space in the inner parishes, as well as the expansion of the suburbs, with subdivision of properties and the construction of small cottages, increasing the numbers of inhabitants and hence of interments. Parishes with small overcrowded churchyards had difficulty finding enough space, especially in an epidemic. During the plague of 1543, the bodies were placed one on the other in the churchyard of St John, Wallbrook, presumably because of lack of room or time to make alternative arrangements, so that the top ones were only eighteen inches below the surface. Shallow burials during the epidemic in 1563 drew a rebuke from the Lord Mayor and the instructions that they should have more earth piled over them, and that all new graves must be of the customary depth.

This problem increased during the second half of the century, exacerbated by the fact that some parishes had taken advantage of the demand for housing by allowing tenements to be built on their churchyards. In response to the plague of 1563, the City set out a new burial ground in 1569 outside Bishopsgate, perhaps on a part of the lands of Bethlem Hospital. Aware that

burial space would not have been available if the epidemic had
continued, it provided the New Churchyard in anticipation of
future need, explaining that 'it is thought good policy to provide for such a lack before the time of necessity requireth it'.
Some parishes also used the churchyard at St Paul's Cathedral
for their burials. This, in turn, had become so full, and some
corpses were at such little depth, that it was almost impossible
to bury the dead satisfactorily and prevent 'putrid exhalations'.
In 1582 the Lord Mayor directed the parishes entitled to use
St Paul's not to do so, instructing them to bury their dead in
the New Churchyard. This did not extend to the interment
of persons of 'honour or worship', but he reduced the number
of parishes authorised to bury there at all from twenty-three
to thirteen.

A respite from the disease after the autumn of 1585 eased
such plague-related problems until they reappeared in 1592.
Simon Forman, physician and astrologer, went to Ipswich in
June, and the day after he returned to London began to develop
the symptoms of plague in his groin; red tokens appeared on
his feet 'as broad as halfpence'. He lanced the buboes himself
as soon as they developed and kept the wounds clean, and
treated himself with 'strong waters' which he had distilled. He
survived, but the effects lingered on and he did not feel well
again for twenty-two weeks. Forman was an early victim of
the outbreak. By mid-August plague was 'dailie increasing' in
London and the Privy Council became concerned, not only
for the implementation of the regulations but because the
outbreak coincided with the return of ships under Martin
Frobisher from a highly successful venture.

The City's merchants had invested £6,000 in the expedition, which intercepted a flotilla of Portuguese vessels returning
from the East Indies, capturing the *Madre de Dios*. This was
said to be the largest ship afloat and richer than 'any shypp
that ever came into England', laden with 537 tons of spices

– the pepper alone was valued at £120,000 – along with cloth, carpets and quilts. For the merchants this was an opportunity not to be missed, and they set off for the West Country ports to buy the cargoes, as well as the jewels plundered by the sailors after the vessel had been captured. They needed to act expeditiously, since the queen claimed the cargo as hers and sent Sir William Cecil with other officials to secure what they could, before other investors took a share, or more of the goods were pilfered. But this produced the danger that they would spread the plague, and so in early September the Council prohibited the merchants from going to Portsmouth, Plymouth or Dartmouth, unless they had a warrant from the Privy Council or the Lord Admiral. The mayors of those towns were instructed to admit only those with such a warrant, wherever they claimed to be from, because the Londoners 'maie disguise themselves and saie they are of other places'. Profit and plague policy came into conflict in this case, but eventually the cargo which remained was taken to London and the vessel itself to Greenwich. The merchants who had supported the venture received twice the value of their investment and so had no great cause to complain of the restrictions. Appropriately enough in the context, some of the profits from the *Madre de Dios* were used towards the cost of building the city's pesthouse, on the north side of the City, in a road that became known as Pest-house Lane, and later Bath Street.

Deaths from plague continued to increase. By the third week of September, almost half of recorded deaths in London were from the disease, although a reassuring letter reported that its victims were mainly in 'the alleys'. The Council wrote to the Lord Mayor and aldermen, complaining of negligence, especially that the sick were not being separated from the healthy, and recommending that the numbers in the prisons be reduced. Some prisoners were being held for minor offences and small debts, which did not justify imprisonment, and the

Council made the obvious point that creditors would do better to come to some arrangement rather than risk losing all of their money if the debtors died.

The outbreak continued into the autumn and so the court came no closer to London than Hampton Court, with access limited to those with licences, and the Law term was held at Hertford Castle. This led to an exchange between the Council and the corporation. The Council was convinced that household quarantine was not being rigorously enforced, that fires in the streets were effective in purging the air and the City's refusal to authorise them was unjustified. It suggested that by not holding the feast and ceremonies at the swearing in of the new Lord Mayor, and applying the money saved towards provisions for those incarcerated in their houses, plague victims would be more willing to observe the quarantine.

The Council also used the transfer of the Law term out of London as an incentive to the City to be more assiduous in enforcing the plague regulations, for it 'must neede turne to the greate hinderaunce of the cittye'. But while holding the courts elsewhere was economically damaging to London, it also created problems, in pushing up prices for accommodation and food in the town where they were held, providing an opportunity which Londoners exploited by moving in to act as suppliers, as well as to attend the hearings. This increased the risk that they would spread the plague. Again, economic opportunities threatened the effectiveness of the policies to contain plague and defeated the object of moving the hearings away from infected places and people. The Lord Mayor responded by submitting suggestions for buildings in London where the courts could be held safely. The Council's response was that this was too late, and the removal of the courts, which the queen was insistent on, could have been prevented by careful execution of the measures to counter the plague. But it did admit that it would have been willing to consider the

City's offer of holding the courts at Guildhall, if it had been made earlier.

Clearly, neither the corporation nor the Council thought that the risk was high in the central areas, despite anxiety that the plague measures were not being effectively applied. In September, the parish of St Margaret, Lothbury appointed two surveyors and the vestry ordered that 'all people kepe the orders sett downe'. Shortly afterwards, eight women were nominated, all pensioners of the parish, who were to 'choose amongest them' which two were to act as searchers, receiving 2s 6d weekly so long as the plague continued. This was as fair a way as any of selecting those who had to carry out that hazardous task; previous experience of diagnosing illnesses was not mentioned. Recorded burials in a sample of twenty-six parishes show that in sixteen of them the number was not significantly above the average, and only in three outer parishes was it more than twice the expected figure. Only St Katherine's-by-the-Tower suffered very high mortality, with a sixfold rise in burials, while the inner parishes escaped relatively lightly and the disease did not spread across the city during 1592.

The number of recorded deaths from plague fell towards the end of the year, but rose again during the middle of January, and the death toll in 1593 was to be far higher than in 1592. Again, stricter enforcement of the existing regulations was the remedy specified by the Privy Council. Quarantined houses were to be locked from the outside and watched, and the occupants were not to be let out until they were free from the disease. Provisions were to be supplied at their own expense unless they were too poor to pay, in which case collections by the City and parishes should be drawn upon. By July, a red cross was being employed as the mark for an infected house, rather than a printed paper, and the Council ordered that it should be nailed to the door, as a painted one could be wiped off. The Council tried to cajole the Lord Mayor and aldermen to enforce the regulations by pointing out that they could be blamed if, for example, the forthcoming meeting of Parliament was not held at Westminster, which would 'greatly prejudice the state of the cittie and people in generall', who might hold them responsible for 'their ruyne'. The warning was a realistic one, for social unrest and anti-alien protests in London had been on the increase in recent years and the Council had complained to the City of the number of disorders.

Yet the difficulties of enforcement remained. Searchers of the dead were appointed by the vestry of St Margaret's, Lothbury in March, but two months later, when the question of inmates was raised, nothing was done and the meeting broke up because 'foulkes would not tary'. Nor would they keep to their houses. In September, Richard Lane of St Margaret's, New Fish Street, 'feeling hymselfe at the begynning of his sicknes weake and faynte', went across the city to visit his aunt, who lived in the parish of St Botolph-without-Aldersgate, half a mile away. His wife was sicker than he was and so both of them should have been confined to their house, but he needed help, for he felt sure that no friends or relatives would visit them because of the plague. He begged his aunt to return with him to nurse them and 'to caste hym in a sweate' to try to cure him. He gave her 6d to pay someone to look after her own affairs and promised that if he and his wife did not survive she would inherit everything. Richard later died and his aunt did claim the inheritance.

Richard was not destitute and his appeal to his aunt to help him with a cure, as well as nursing care, may have been because he was unable to find a doctor to treat him, rather than his inability to pay one. Simon Forman remained through- out the outbreak, despite suffering from plague the previous year, and noted that the 'Doctors all did fly', while he stayed to care for the 'distressed poor'. From his experiences he produced *A Discourse of the Plague*, more useful to its readers for its description of the disease and methods of treatment than for his explanation of its causes, which he discussed in terms of divine punishment for wickedness.

But the government was convinced that the disease could be transmitted, from person to person directly, or indirectly by textiles, as illustrated in an account sent to Sir Robert Cecil, the acting Secretary of State. This related the experiences of two brothers who took a boat from Greenwich to London. One of them fell sick that evening and his life was despaired of, but he took some medicine and recovered. His brother had a slight headache and did not feel unwell enough to need any treatment until five days later, when the 'marks' appeared in his neck and so he took to his bed. On the following day he drank eight or nine jugs of cold drink, presumably hoping to cleanse himself, but he died. The waterman and their landlady were also taken ill. The explanation offered was that it was a wet day when they travelled and, as the waterman had no awning for the boat, they sheltered beneath a bed cover that had been on the bed of someone who had died of the plague, and they had contracted the disease from that.

By the summer, business was said to have come to a standstill, and a merchant in Hull, afraid to return to London while the epidemic continued, commented ironically that only a cargo of onions and garlic would be profitable. Because of their strong taste and smell, both were thought to help keep the plague at bay. Edward Alleyn repeated the advice of contemporary authors when he wrote from Bristol to his wife, at their house in Bankside, that she should 'kepe it fayr and clean', throw water outside the door and in the back yard every evening and in the windows put 'good store of rwe and herbe of grace'. Philip Henslow was afraid because plague had claimed victims all around, in 'all moste every howsse'. At the end of September, he had to report that almost all of his neighbours had died and that his two servant girls had contracted the plague, but had recovered. His news of business was also bad, for although Bartholomew's Fair had been held, he had not sold Alleyn's horse because he was offered such a low price, and 'as for your tenenantes we cane geat no Rent'. The Privy Council had directed that the fair should not be held and, when the Lord Mayor had protested, it had used the threat of cancellation as an incentive to the City to enforce the plague regulations. It eventually relented and the fair did take place, but lasted just three days and was for wholesale goods only.

In such circumstances, collection of rates and taxes was difficult. The vestry at St Margaret's, Lothbury ordered that a monthly rate should be collected as long as the epidemic lasted, to pay the searchers, increased to four, and those who were quarantined and unable to support themselves. But some parishioners did not pay, perhaps because they were absent, and almost a fifth of the amount due was not received. Voluntary donations were therefore a vital element in providing for the sick poor. The parish received £2 13s 10d from 'sondry persons', £2 of which came from one donor. All levies were likely to be difficult during the epidemic and yet, despite its policies to contain the plague, in July the Privy Council sent an order for the enlistment of 200 soldiers to serve in Normandy. When the Common Council asked for a reduction because of the epidemic, the Council agreed that they could be drawn from elsewhere, on condition that London paid the costs, including coats and weapons. To cover the outlay, the Common Council imposed a rate, but this was a low priority at such a time and the money was never collected.

Other places took care to prevent the epidemic spreading. Winchester's Common Council issued an order that no one coming from an infected place should be allowed into the city and anyone who had arrived already was to be expelled forthwith. Even someone from a place free from the plague could stay only one night. A watch was set at the city's gates to restrict admission. Yet in September one of the aldermen was discovered to have ignored the order and gone to London, 'in this danger of Infection, and there boughte and retaylled Wares'. His need to continue trading in London was so compelling that he ignored both the risk of contracting plague there and the orders of his own city's government, of which he was a senior member. He was condemned to fourteen days' imprisonment, and if he refused to comply his shop window was to be shut down and he prohibited from trading for one month.

The epidemic in 1593 was the worst since 1563, with burials 4.25 times higher than in a normal year. But the distribution of deaths contrasted with that in 1563, with the heaviest mortality in 1593 in the parishes around the City, which escaped relatively lightly. The experience of the richer central parishes in 1593 may reflect the comparatively high proportion of parishioners who could leave during the epidemic, and perhaps more effective enforcement of the regulations in those small parishes than in the larger and increasingly populous ones fringing the City. But they did not escape the experiences typical of a plague epidemic. At St Mary's, Aldermary, two sisters, servants to Edward Breth, were buried on the same day in July, and the register records the burial a week later of Sara Hering 'which died in the street of the plague'. St Peter's, Cornhill lost one of its respected parishioners, Robert Salisbury, an upholsterer and 'an upright and just man', and his ten-year-old son, who was buried in the same grave.

Among the outer parishes, St James', Clerkenwell experienced a fourfold increase in burials compared with the early years of the decade, and at St Martin's—in-the-Fields there was a threefold increase. In the crowded north-east parishes of St Botolph-without-Aldgate and St Botolph-without-Bishopsgate, the numbers of burials were six times higher than normal, and St Katherine's-by-the-Tower suffered even more heavily than in the previous year and was by far the worst affected of a sample of twenty-two parishes. St Botolph's recorded only thirty-eight burials of plague victims in 1592, but in 1593 the figure was 1,078. Far more males died than females – of the plague burials in 1593, 604 were males and 474 were females – and there was a distinct pattern to the age of the victims, with comparatively few parishioners over forty years old dying of plague. However, the balance between the sexes may reflect the composition of the population of that parish on the eve of the epidemic, rather than a greater susceptibility to plague among males, for a wider sample of parishes shows that the numbers of male and female burials were more or less equal. On the other hand, analysis of the ages at death in St Peter's, Cornhill and Allhallows, London Wall confirms that those over twenty and, even more, those over forty were less susceptible than children over five years old and teenagers.

When Joan Alleyn wrote to her husband in August, she was unable to give an accurate figure for the numbers of deaths, but thought that the weekly death toll from all causes was 1,700 or 1,800. She implied that there was an attempt to suppress the information, telling her husband that 'I cane not seand you no Juste note of yt be cause there is command ment to the contrary', and her estimate seems too high when compared with the total mortality. The number of deaths for the year entered by the clerk of St Peter's, Cornhill in the parish register was 25,886, of which the plague accounted for 15,003. He then added a personal note:

In a thousand five hundred ninety and three
The Lord preserved my house and mee
When of pestilence theare died
Full manie a thousand els beeside

His figure was for the whole of London and suggests a death rate of almost thirteen per cent; within the City and the liberties the number of deaths between 21 December 1592 and 20 December 1593 was 17,844, with 10,662 of them attributed to plague.

By January 1594, the epidemic was almost over. It had been a test for the policies designed to deal with plague and the experience had not caused any essential alteration to them, but had reinforced some opinions. When Burghley introduced a Bill into the House of Lords to limit further building in London, he made the connection once more between overcrowding and plague. From the limited beginnings early in the century, the government had evolved a coherent policy to combat plague. Confident in the efficacy of its policies, its main efforts became directed towards their enforcement rather than their development, which in London meant ensuring that the rules were applied rigorously enough to be effective, working through the Lord Mayor and aldermen and, as the population beyond their jurisdiction expanded, the justices of the peace for Middlesex and Surrey.

Although the outbreak in 1592–93 produced little change to the policies aimed at tackling the problem of the disease, it did contribute to the sense of gloom which hung over the closing decade of the century, and plague again caused the closure of the playhouses in 1596. Foreign wars, the rebellion in Ireland and lingering uncertainties about the Protestant succession added to problems caused by poor harvests and high food prices, trade dislocation and social unrest. Plague had become linked with public hygiene, poor housing, overcrowding, vagrancy and disorder, as well as heightening the tension between civic and national government and being a focus of stress between the wealthy and the urban poor.

3

The Plague in Early Stuart London

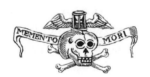

In 1603 Elizabeth died and was succeeded by James VI of
Scotland. The transition from the old reign and dynasty
to the new one went smoothly, despite fears of disorder.
The long-standing uncertainties over the succession had been
resolved without difficulty, for the new monarch, James I of
England, was married with two sons, and he was a Protestant.
He came to the throne on the death of Elizabeth on 24 March
and reached London in May, going first to the Charterhouse
on the northern edge of the City, as Elizabeth had done thirty-
five years earlier. As part of the welcoming ceremonies for

the king, the corporation planned a pageant and commissioned Thomas Dekker to write a panegyric for it. In his *The Magnificent Entertainment*, Dekker developed the idea of the new king coming from the clean air of the north to disperse the miasma which threatened to bring plague.

Stimulating northerly winds were commonly believed to be healthier than southerly ones, which brought the warm air that created the conditions for a plague epidemic. Windows facing the north and east should be kept open during the daytime when the air was clear, although not, of course, if unsavoury smells such as those from fogs or dunghills could waft in. A north wind would dry all infected vapours, and so orientation had to be taken into consideration when treatment for those infected was being arranged. A hospital for the sick should face north-east, so that it was open to the north wind and would not be too hot in summer.

Unfortunately, the spring of 1603 was a warm one, increasing the apprehension of an outbreak of plague, and early in March the fear was expressed that the year would be 'very contagious'. Shortly afterwards, the Privy Council closed all English ports as the queen's health deteriorated, although as one of the measures to ensure a smooth succession rather than part of the attempts to prevent plague from reaching London. But the Lord Mayor acted on his own initiative and on 12 April asked for an order to prevent plays being performed, and requested that the justices for Surrey and Middlesex should be alerted to the danger and instructed to implement the customary regulations. He saw the suburbs, especially Whitechapel, Clerkenwell and Shoreditch, as 'more subiecte to the Infection then any other Places' and by 5 April the aldermen were aware of plague deaths around Kentish Street in Southwark. This was an early response to the danger and one that had not been prompted solely by the numbers of plague deaths which were being returned by the parish clerks.

Their figures were, in any case, treated with a degree of scepticism. By 1584, the corporation was alert to the fact that not all those who died of plague showed the symptoms and that there was some deliberate under-recording, because 'sometime fraude of the searchers may deceive'. Moreover, no record was kept of those who contracted the disease and recovered. Rather than rely on the cause of death as set down, they had adopted the simple rule that when the number of deaths exceeded fifty per week, which they observed to be the norm, plague was responsible. Almost twenty years later, the population had increased and the number of deaths was commensurately higher, roughly 100 per week. But in the four weeks before the Lord Mayor made his request, only 312 burials were recorded, with just fifteen of the deaths attributed to plague. It is clear that the returns of burials, which were designed to alert the authorities to the beginnings of an epidemic, had not been the sole cause of the corporation's concern on this occasion, and it had reacted to other information, perhaps from the parish officers, from experience and in the context of outbreaks on the continent.

The disease had been widespread in northern Europe in recent years; 1601, 1602 and 1603 were plague years in both Amsterdam and Rotterdam. The epidemic in Amsterdam in 1602 was especially bad and the Privy Council acted in July to prevent anyone from there landing in London, at the ports on the Thames or those around the south-east coast. Travellers who had disembarked already were to be treated almost as if they were cargo and sent out of the towns to camp in the fields for forty days. By September, plague was rife in Great Yarmouth and the Lord Mayor issued an order prohibiting contact with Yarmouth and Amsterdam. Despite the precautions, in October two houses in Wapping, where goods from Danzig had been taken in, were reported to have been infected with plague and all of their occupants were said to have died of the disease. Lord Cobham, Lord Warden of the Cinque Ports, warned that unless especial care was taken there would be a plague epidemic in England in the following year. A further risk came from contacts with the Dutch garrison of Ostend, which was besieged by the Spanish armies for no less than 167 weeks between July 1601 and September 1604. In September 1601, there were over 4,500 English soldiers in the garrison, although the number was later reduced, and from May 1602 plague was killing between sixty and eighty victims in the town every day, and was still active there early in 1603.

The danger was all the greater because of the king's Scottish entourage coming from Edinburgh, which was experiencing an outbreak, and the sheer numbers of people who came to London at the start of the new reign, to establish themselves at James' court or simply to witness the coronation, appropriately fixed for St James' Day, 25 July. Giovanni Scaramelli, the Venetian Secretary in England, believed that by then there would be an extra 100,000 extra mouths to feed in the capital, and that already more than 40,000 gentlemen had arrived. The warm weather persisted and in the middle of May he began to report the numbers both of plague deaths and of parishes affected. The corporation's judgement was shown to have been correct and Dekker's choice of theme singularly unfortunate, for the number of plague deaths, which averaged just over five a week during March and April, grew steadily during the early summer, so that the City's pageant could not be performed.

The king was sufficiently alarmed to order that those who had come to London should leave at the end of the term, partly because the risk of the plague spreading was increased 'by concourse of people abiding there'. The number of infected parishes rose steadily, from six to thirteen before the end of May and to seventeen by the middle of June, but even then only forty-three deaths from the disease were recorded in the weekly Bill. But the customary orders had been issued, directing that a printed paper inscribed with 'Lord, have mercy upon us' be fixed to the door of an infected house, and that stray dogs should be killed. The dog catcher at St Margaret's, Westminster reacted dutifully to the latter order and claimed for 502 dogs killed in the parish during the epidemic.

In early July, plague deaths had reached seventy-two in thirty parishes, and in Westminster nine houses had been isolated as infected, in which eleven people had died, seven of them women. The intervals between deaths in single houses justified a long period of quarantine, for in a house in Thieving Lane the two deaths from plague were separated by fourteen days and in Longditch a plague death on 18 June was followed by another in the same house on 1 July. These were not high numbers, but the court remained out of London nevertheless. Scaramelli reported that the possibility of either advancing or postponing the date of the coronation had been discussed. The decision was taken for it to go ahead as planned, but without the royal progress through the city or the 'Shewes and Ornaments' that had been prepared for the occasion. A royal proclamation made it clear that the rising number of plague deaths was the reason for the cancellation of the accustomed ceremonial, and expressed the government's fear of both an increase of the disease in London because of the crowds and its spread throughout the country when the visitors returned home.

The sense of anticlimax and disappointment was expressed by Gilbert Dugdale. Londoners had welcomed the new king, 'which hour of glory was dashed by the omnipotency of God's power; who, mortally visiting the City and land with a general Visitation, hath, since that time, taken thousands to his mercy'. The frustration was increased by the economic effects of the epidemic, especially the check which it gave to those trades that had begun to benefit from an upsurge in business accompanying the feeling of expectation which followed the king's accession and the influx of visitors, especially those preening themselves before they appeared at court.

Action to stem the outbreak had been taken at an early stage, but was shown to be futile as the numbers of plague deaths continued to increase. This was an embarrassment to the Privy Council and the City at the start of the new reign. Not only had it not ushered in the healthy and prosperous times described by Dekker, but the Stuart dynasty, like the Tudor one, was inaugurated with a devastating epidemic. James might have expected more stringent measures to have been taken, in line with those enforced at Edinburgh, and Scaramelli, familiar with Venice's rigorous arrangements, certainly thought that the City's response was somewhat sluggish. But one improvement which was introduced was the inclusion of figures for the eight outer parishes and the pesthouse in the Bills of Mortality. This was first done for the week ending 21 July, raising the numbers of deaths sharply, from 612 to 1,186 and plague deaths from 434 to 917. In the week before the change, plague deaths were sixty-nine per cent of the total, but when the outer parishes were included they were seventy-seven per cent, supporting the Lord Mayor's contention that the suburbs were suffering relatively badly. With their inclusion, the Bills gave a more realistic indication of the situation in the capital, but they were still incomplete, omitting Westminster, the Savoy, Newington, Islington, Lambeth and Hackney.

The pesthouse made only a small difference to the numbers. From its inclusion until the end of December, only 135 people were recorded as dying there, suggesting that it was far too small to be of much value in isolating the sick during a major epidemic. The cost of maintaining someone there may also have limited the numbers admitted. In July, the Court of Aldermen ordered that those who were sent to the pesthouse should be maintained by the householder or the parish, with an initial payment of 13s 4d towards 'surgery, women keepers, and other extraordinary charges'. The City itself had contributed £115 for bedding, medicine and other items by 13 September. Moreover, the staff at the pesthouse had the reputation of being neglectful and even cruel, which was a strong disincentive to sending a relative there.

The corporation distributed printed copies of the plague orders among the parishes on 12 July and the usual measures were put in place. St James's Fair in Westminster was cancelled on 9 July, and not only St Bartholomew's Fair but all other fairs within fifty miles of London were banned by an order of 8 August, and the Michaelmas Law term was adjourned to Winchester. The central, wealthier, parishes were able to manage the crisis effectively. The vestry of St Michael's Cornhill built a shed as an addition to the parish pesthouse and sent 'diverse poore' there for treatment, donated 4d daily to each of the victims and paid for the burials of the poor who died of the disease. The parish sexton received 6d daily for checking that the poor victims and vagrants did not 'wandr about the stretes'. But in the larger parishes around the fringes of the City, some problems which had arisen in earlier epidemics reappeared, and as the numbers of those infected increased, the arrangements for supplying them with provisions proved inadequate. The poorer parishes were the worst affected, because 'where the infection most rageth there povertie raigneth among the commons, which having no supplies to satisfie the greedie desire of those that should attend them, are for the most part left desolate & die without reliefe'.

As early as the middle of July, there was alarm that the disease would continue to spread, as the poor would not comply with the orders. In St Martin's-in-the-Fields, those who should have been quarantined had to be forced into their houses, and the printed papers on the doors were pulled off, so that the infected houses could not be identified. Stricter punishments were requested for those who would not remain indoors or tore down the papers. But enforcement was difficult, especially where there was inadequate supervision. Some 'gracelesse and Lawlesse' people ignored or even resisted the regulations and would not 'Endure ther dores wher the sicknesse ys to be shutt up'. According to Dekker, some tried to avoid having their houses closed by taking away bodies surreptitiously, 'least the fatall hand-writing of death should seal up their doores'. If this was reprehensible, so was the reaction of those wealthy householders who refused to pay a rate to support those who were immured.

One of Sir Robert Cecil's correspondents found the conditions in the area between the City and Westminster to be deplorable. A bowling alley and an alehouse next to it were the resort of all kinds of people, who mixed together regardless of the risk of plague, even on Sundays. Carpenters working at Worcester House lodged elsewhere in the city and came from their lodgings daily to work, despite the fact that some had died there of the plague. And other regulations were ignored, with pigs freely scavenging in the streets and too many dogs kept in small houses. Only one justice of the peace was at hand to try to control such dangerous practices, and not only was he 'a sickly man', but his authority did not extend beyond the Savoy to the other liberties.

At the end of August, Sir William Waad, a clerk of the Privy Council, confirmed that a part of the problem was that the Middlesex justices with jurisdiction within London had left, and so had the aldermen and 'better sort', who had moved from the city to the country. Many of the poorer people, too, went away, some to nearby villages, where the constables, fearful for their own safety, would not take any action against them. Those who could not find lodgings slept in barns or under the hedges. Waad wrote from his own experiences at Hampstead, where the sick from London were dying in yards and outhouses. Within the city, the streets were strewn with straw, bedding, mats and rags, in clear defiance of the regulations. He complained that without the presence of the aldermen and justices such behaviour could not be prevented, because the junior officers were 'not regarded'. But he also admitted that it was easier to object to these actions than to prevent them.

Funerals had also attracted his attention, for he was aware that they were being conducted as if conditions were normal, and with less solemnity than was appropriate. The streets were strewn with flowers when girls or spinsters were buried and at a bachelor's funeral the mourners wore rosemary, as if they were at a marriage. A more pertinent objection was that funerals brought people together in groups, increasing the danger of plague being spread. In May, the corporation issued an order changing its policy on interments, now ruling that plague victims were to be buried only during the night, not before ten o'clock, and the Lord Mayor also issued precepts complaining of the 'multitudes' following the dead to the grave and ordering that the number at a funeral should not exceed six. The City Marshal attempted to enforce these regulations, arresting offenders and imprisoning them. But he was not supported by the clergy, who, rather than reproving those at a funeral for attending, told the marshal that this was within the bishop's jurisdiction, not his. He also met with more forceful objections and on one occasion, when trying to turn back those in 'a great multitude' following a corpse to the burial ground, he and his two men were beaten up.

Resentment at someone in authority intervening at such a sensitive time was coupled with an awareness that, in reality, not all of those who gathered in groups at a funeral, in an alehouse or elsewhere would die. When Sir Walter Raleigh was taken from the Tower on 12 November, on his way to his trial at Winchester, fifty horsemen were required to escort him through the 'multitudes of unruly people'. Those who had assembled to jeer the unpopular favourite of Elizabeth,

now fallen so far as to be accused of treason, seemingly had no
fear of mixing promiscuously in a large throng, even though
545 deaths had been recorded during the previous week.
Furthermore, from their experiences in the current epidemic
and from the collective memory of past outbreaks, Londoners
were aware that some of those who came into direct contact
with the sick and their possessions survived. Nurses appointed
by the parishes and those who, from duty to a relative or out of
neighbourliness, looked after the victims did not all succumb
to the disease. And many who were incarcerated in houses that
were closed and guarded by the parish officers, and in which
there were deaths, nevertheless emerged alive from the ordeal.
The policies to control plague were based on the belief that the
disease was infectious, but the population was not convinced.
The point was made by Dekker, who posed the question,

> Can we believe that one mans breath
> Infected, and being blowne from him,
> His poyson should to others swim:
> For then who breath'd upon the first?
> Where did th'imbulked venome burst?
> Or how scapte those that did divide
> The self-same bits with those that dide?
> Drunke of the self-same cups, and laie
> In Ulcerous beds, as close as they?

His observations are confirmed by the parish registers, which
show that in 1603, as in other outbreaks, some households
suffered multiple deaths, but that they were not typical. A
household in St Helen's, Bishopsgate lost three family members and three servants in September, yet in the majority of
households in that parish there was only one death.

Dekker also mocked the notion that textiles carried the
disease and should be avoided. He wrote, in an ironic tone,

that the infection 'loved to be lapt warme, and lie smothring in a shag-hayrde Rugge, or an old fashionde Coverlid'. And so people would not go into upholsterers' shops, among their dangerous rugs and featherbeds, and would cover their faces when they went past the woollen drapers' shops along Watling Street. The conviction that sweet smells gave protection was also ridiculed by Dekker, with a description of a coach which was driven through London. He may have seen it himself, for he commented that he had noted down the date, 9 August: 'This fearefull pittifull Coach was all hung with Rue from the top to the toe of the Boote, to keepe the leather and the nayles from infection; the very Nosthrills of the Coach-horses were stopt with hearb-grace, that I pittied the poore beasts being almost windlesse.' Yet they ran through Cornhill 'as if the Divell had bene Coachman'. Someone desperately anxious to ward off the disease had put their faith in 'good' odours and speed of travel.

Such fears surely were fallacious if, as the government as well as the Church pronounced, God sent epidemics and controlled their severity and duration. In June, a royal proc-lamation acknowledged that the disease would end 'through the mercifull goodness of Almighty God' and another, in September, referred to the outbreak as one 'which Almighty God would cease at his good pleasure'. The opening of James' first Parliament was delayed until March 1604 because of the epidemic, and in the speech from the throne the king explained that, 'It did no sooner please God to lighten his hand, and relent the violence of his devouring Angel against the poore people of this Citie, but as soone did I resolve to call this Parliament.' Such pronouncements were common and, taken at their face value in a society in which belief in God was unquestioned, at least outwardly, and not interpreted as conventional expressions of piety, then God did play the cen-tral role in plague epidemics. And if the disease came by the hand of God and was halted by him, it followed that it was not contagious. According to James Balmford's experience in Southwark in 1603, that opinion was 'stiffely maintained' by many, including some of the 'better sort'.

Balmford was one of the London clergy faced with the difficult task of reconciling the two points of view, maintaining that plague was a punishment for sin and that the outbreak would abate when society had been chastised for its errors, yet insisting that the regulations imposed by the magistrates should be observed. But Henoch Clapham did not follow his fellow clergymen, who were endeavouring to support those policies, and he believed that the outbreak could be explained in terms of divine providence. Preservation came through faith, not medicines. Plague victims died because their hour had come; taking care by avoiding others was pointless, and attending church and following a body to the grave in a crowd of mourners did not increase the risk of contracting the disease. He expressed his views in *An Epistle discoursing upon the present Pestilence: teaching what it is, and how the people of God should carrie themselves towards God and their Neighbour herein*, but it was perhaps more through his sermons that he represented an immediate challenge to the official point of view. Attendance at church services was high, and a persuasive preacher had a wider and more direct influence than the magistrates, and commanded respect for remaining when they and others in authority had gone.

The underlying tension between belief and regulations had not been so evident before 1603. Clapham played a major role in bringing the issue to the fore, and did appear to be influential. His views were repeated, and the marshal blamed him for encouraging those who continued to go to funerals and oppose his authority. On 13 November, Clapham was taken into custody for criticising the plague orders and was kept in prison until the following August, which reduced his own influence during the epidemic but could not suppress the conviction, reported by a Spanish visitor to London in 1609, that the victims were those who had been singled out by God. Conversely, those who did their duty were not harmed. The Dutch merchant and writer Jacob Cool remained in London throughout 1603 and a friend wrote from Middelburg to commend him for having done so, adding that he did not doubt that God had rewarded him by sparing his family and restoring a relative to good health. Even so, the epidemic was a dreadful experience for Cool, who wrote an account of it, in which he stressed that he would never be able to forget the sense of grief that pervaded the city and that what he had seen had caused even his courage to falter.

Unlike Cool, Lancelot Andrewes, Dean of Westminster, rector of St Giles-in-the-Fields and soon to be appointed as bishop of Chichester, had left London during the outbreak. Clapham was questioned by Andrewes, and the recantation which was presented for him to sign included a justification for such action in the statement that 'a faithful Christian man, whether magistrate or minister, may in such times hide or withdraw himself, as well corporeally as spiritually, and use local flight to a more healthful place (taking sufficient order for the discharge of his function)'. Andrewes clearly felt the need to exonerate his own actions, but such a view would not have been widely shared among those who had remained. Dekker satirised the exodus of the leading citizens by describing 'this pestiferous shipwrack of Londoners, when the Pilot, Boatswains, Maister and Maister's-mates, with all the chiefe Mariners that had charge in this goodly Argozy of government, leapt from the sterne... crying out onely, Put your trust in God my Bullies, & not in us', and either hid under hatches or made their way ashore in the boats. Nor did he spare those parish officers who remained, and strictly applied the orders, condemning the constables for 'charging poore sick

wretches that had neither meate nor mony, in the kings name
to keepe their houses, that's to say, to famish & die'.

These tensions and controversies were set against the background of rising mortality in the worst epidemic since 1563.
By the beginning of August, deaths exceeded 2,000 in one
week, and a fortnight later they had risen to more than 3,000.
For five weeks, from the middle of August, the weekly number
of deaths ranged between 2,853 and 3,385, with eighty-nine
per cent of them recorded as being from plague. Not until
the third week of October was the total number of deaths
below 1,000, and it was another month before it fell to fewer
than 500. As the number of deaths declined, so did the proportion of those from plague, but even in November they
still constituted seventy-five per cent of the total. During
the year, plague deaths accounted for eighty-one per cent of
the 43,154 recorded burials. This total includes Westminster,
Lambeth, Stepney, Hackney, Islington, Newington Butts and
the Savoy, but not the eight out-parishes and seven outer districts, and some Londoners died elsewhere. The true figures
were, therefore, somewhat higher, and the total population of
London is uncertain, but an estimate that twenty per cent of
its inhabitants died during the epidemic cannot be far wide
of the mark.

The variation in the social impact of the epidemic observed
in earlier outbreaks was commented on again. James Balmford
blamed the extent of the disaster on the overcrowding in the
poorer areas, where the houses and alleys 'did vomit out their
undigested dead, Who by cartloads are carried to their grave;
For all those lanes with folk were overfed'. The outer parishes
were those which were most badly affected, while the area
around Cheapside suffered proportionately less. The highest
mortality was in St Olave's, Southwark, St Giles, Cripplegate
and St Sepulchre's, while in Allhallows, London Wall the
number of deaths was more than ten times the norm, and in

St Botolph's-without-Bishopsgate it was almost nine times. Even so, the inner City parishes did not escape lightly in real terms. In the small parish of St Leonard's Eastcheap, which covered less than one-and-a-half acres, the register records seventy burials in 1603, three more than in the epidemic year of 1563, and more than five times the average for the years 1602–11. And, as Jacob Cool suggested, the balance of recorded deaths between the inner and outer parishes might have been distorted by householders in the central area sending their sick servants to their 'garden- or pleasure-houses' in the suburban parishes, where they died. Dekker alleged that the City trades-men dispatched their servants who were plague victims in sacks from their houses to those of their outworkers who lived in the suburbs, so that the deaths were recorded there and their own houses and shops were not closed. The outworkers were afraid to refuse, fearing economic retribution by the withdrawal of work, which would lead to their 'utter undoing'.

Cool also noted that the recruitment of nurses, watchmen and searchers became easier as the numbers who found them-selves out of work increased. Perhaps, too, fear of the disease declined during the outbreak despite its virulence. According to Dekker, some who were infected recovered, to go about their business 'with sounder limmes, than many who came out of France, and the Netherlands', which he evidently regarded as the source of the epidemic. From the relative safety of Sunbury-upon-Thames, Giovanni Scaramelli commented in August that many of the sick recovered. But others did not. Ben Jonson's seven-year-old son Benjamin died of the plague. Lea Barker, a twenty-one-year-old merchant's daughter of St Peter's, Cornhill, was taken ill on her wedding day in August and died five days later. And some suffered such hideous deaths that the fears of those who were caring for them would have been heightened rather than assuaged. Simon Forman's only son, Joshua, was taken ill on a Sunday in early October and died on the following Saturday. He developed an abscess in his stomach and red marks in his groin, described by Forman as 'tokens'. When the abscess burst, he 'vomited a great bellyfull' and then suffered repeated bouts of vomiting, dying 'with his fingers in his mouth'.

Joshua was eighteen-and-a-half when he died; as in earlier plague epidemics, a high proportion of the victims were children and young adults. Before 1603, those aged between five and twenty-four in St Botolph's-without-Bishopsgate accounted for thirteen per cent of burials, but during the outbreak they were forty-five per cent of the total, and in Allhallows, London Wall the number of children who died was more than twenty times the average. In thirty-two households in St Helen's, Bishopsgate, from the end of May until late August, nineteen of the forty-five people who died were children and a further eighteen were described as servants, many of whom may have been adolescents or young adults. In February 1604, it was pointed out that because of the numbers of apprentices and servants who had died, 'divers masters, householders, and shopkeepers do want apprentices and servants'. This is confirmed by the numbers of new apprentices enrolled, which increased by seventy-four per cent in the two years following the epidemic.

Their deaths contributed to the disruption of the normal working patterns in the city. In the middle of October 1603, Scaramelli reported to Venice that all public and private affairs were 'in absolute confusion'. None would pay their debts, in the hope that their creditors would soon die and payment could therefore be avoided, and orders placed with the merchants were cancelled. French importers of English broadcloth were reluctant to receive any shipments because of the plague. Although the English authorities argued that it was not prevalent in all of the producing areas, London's role as the centre of cloth finishing seriously affected the industry while the plague raged there. Shortcloth exports from London were down by one-third in 1603.

Customs and taxes could not be collected in the capital, which paid such a high proportion of the revenue from taxation that the treasury's receipts fell and its reserves were depleted as a result. Collection of a triple subsidy voted by Parliament in 1601 was incomplete when Elizabeth died, with at least £200,000 outstanding. But the City merchants told the king that the plague had brought trade to a standstill, and they could not meet his request for a loan, even when he dropped his requirement from £40,000 to £10,000. Their reply reflected the reality of the situation – they were scattered and the practicalities of tax collection would be difficult in a city disrupted by plague – but it did not help to create good relations between the Crown and the City at this early stage of the new reign.

As the number of deaths declined in the winter, the problems decreased and London's life returned to normal. In March, Parliament assembled, and the king at last made his entry into the city on 15 March, processing with his entourage from the Tower to Westminster. The crowds who came to watch the procession did not produce any great increase in the numbers of plague deaths, and by July the Venetian ambassador could describe London as 'the healthiest place in the kingdom'. The plague had struck many English towns during 1603 and the outbreak continued to claim victims throughout 1604. London's death rate had indeed fallen sharply, but the ambassador's confidence was misplaced, because the disease did not entirely subside, as it commonly did after an epidemic year, and 896 of the 5,219 deaths recorded in London in 1604 were from plague. The situation during the summer was serious enough for the corporation to consider cancelling Bartholomew Fair, although after some vacillation it did allow it to go ahead, on 27 August.

Such uncertainty, produced by the numbers of plague deaths, continued for several years, but without a large-scale epidemic developing. When John Graunt examined the statistics from the Bills, in the 1660s, he concluded that 'the plague of 1603 lasted eight Years', because only in 1605 did the number of plague deaths fall below 500; in the next three years they exceeded 2,000, in 1609 as many as 4,240 were recorded as dying from the disease, and in 1610 the number was 1,803. A royal proclamation in September 1609 described the plague as being 'dispersed in divers of the best and most open streets', and in the week ending 21 September plague deaths numbered 240, the highest weekly figure for the whole period. Parliament's scheduled sitting in November was postponed until the following February because of the outbreak. September and October were the most pestilent months in every year during this sequence, except for 1610, when the peak came slightly earlier, in the last week of August.

The area included in the Bills of Mortality was enlarged in 1604, with the addition of parishes in Westminster, around the City to the north and east, Bermondsey, and Bridewell, and from 1606 the Savoy was included. Also reassessed in the light of the experiences of 1603 were the administration of the pesthouse and the charges which were to be levied there. The admission charge was set at 10s and the daily fees for a poor person came to 1s 2d, including food, lodging, medical and nursing care, with an extra 2d daily for fuel during the six winter months. And so the cost of keeping someone there for four weeks during those months was £2 7s 4d.

The interrelated problems of providing for those who were isolated in their houses and enforcing the quarantine were addressed in an Act of Parliament in 1604, 'for the charitable relief and ordering of persons infected with the plague'. The Act acknowledged that poor people could not be provided for by their fellow citizens during epidemics, and that some

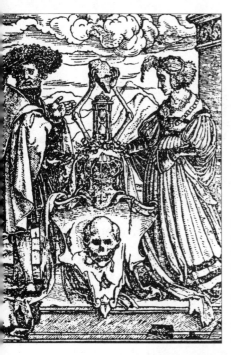

1 Images of death were a recurrent theme in European art, stimulated by the high mortality during the periodic plague epidemics, and the foulness of the disease. This allegorical escutcheon of death by Hans Holbein the younger contains the characteristic motifs of a skull, a skeleton and an hourglass.

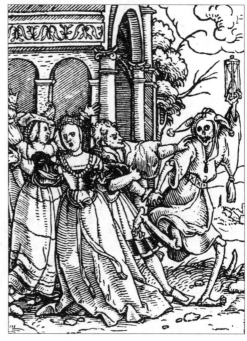

2 Plague was an indiscriminate killer, sparing none. Here Death pursues the queen and her entourage, in a scene from Holbein's *Dance of Death* (c. 1523–26).

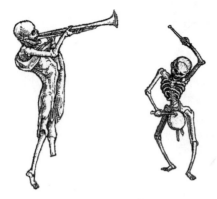

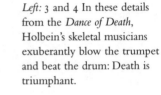

Left: 3 and 4 In these details from the *Dance of Death*, Holbein's skeletal musicians exuberantly blow the trumpet and beat the drum: Death is triumphant.

Below left: 5 A skeleton carrying the arrow of death and a spade for burials precedes an angel of death, who has an hourglass and scythe, in this illustration from a broadsheet of 1577.

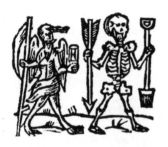

Below: 6 Sixteenth-century London was largely concentrated on the north side of the River Thames, within the medieval city walls.

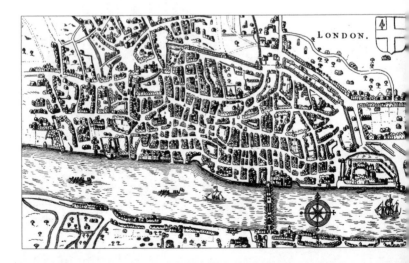

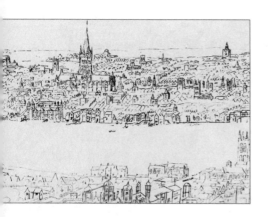

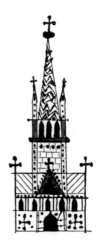

Above left: 7 This section of Anthonis van den Wyngaerde's pen-and-ink drawing of *c.*1544 is dominated by St Paul's cathedral, with its tall spire. In the foreground is Southwark, on the south side of the Thames, with the tower of the church of St Mary Overy on the extreme right.

Above right: 8 The west front of St Paul's, redrawn from an early fourteenth-century manuscript describing the foundation of the city. The ornate spire was destroyed by fire in 1561 and not rebuilt.

Below: 9 Wyngaerde's view of London from Southwark shows the densely packed buildings running back from the wharves at Billingsgate to the church of St Mary Spital. The prominent tower and spire in the centre of this view are those of the church of St Dunstan-in-the-East.

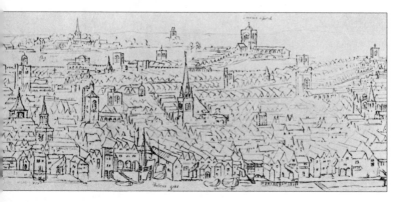

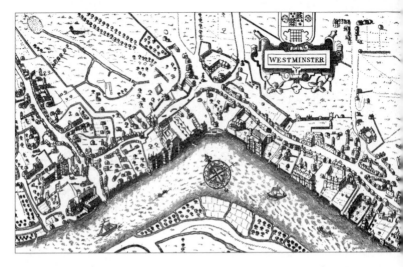

10 To the west of the City, a ribbon-development of houses and palaces led to Charing Cross, in the centre of this plan, and continued to Westminster, with its abbey church and royal palace.

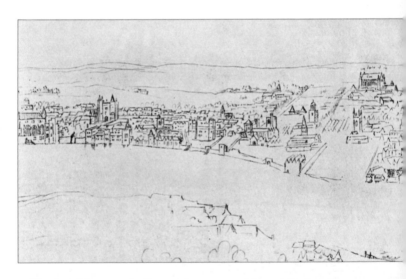

11 The Strand, between Ludgate, at the extreme right, and Durham House, lined with aristocratic mansions and bishops' palaces. The pinnacled tower is the gateway to the Savoy hospital and the prominent church to the right, without a spire or tower, is the chapel of Ely House.

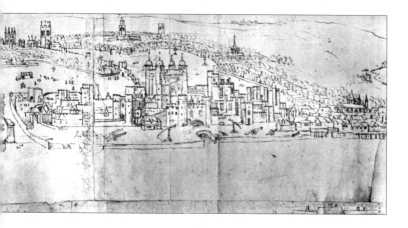

12 The Tower of London and Tower Wharf and, beyond them, Whitechapel and East Smithfield, already a growing and crowded suburb when Wyngaerde made his drawing c.1544. The churches of St Botolph-without-Aldgate and the Minories are on the skyline on the left of this section of his view.

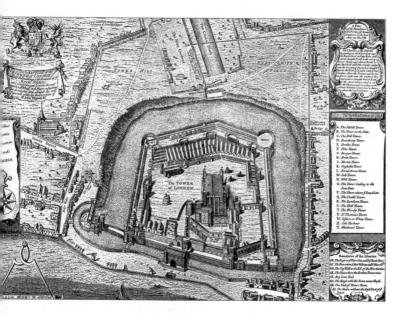

13 The Tower c.1597, still very much a fortress, walled and moated, from where Sir Walter Raleigh was taken for his trial during the plague outbreak in 1603.

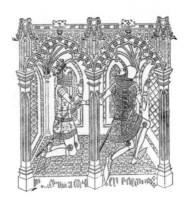

14 The Black Death reached England in 1348, during the reign of Edward III. In this drawing of a wall painting in St Stephen's chapel, Westminster, the king and St George are shown praying. St Stephen's was destroyed by fire in 1834.

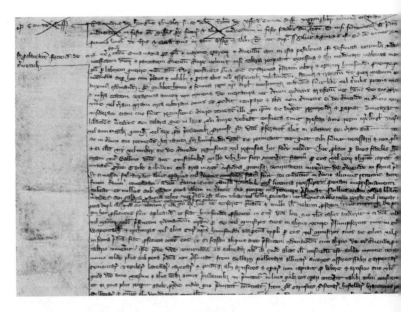

15 The Black Death may have killed as many as one-third of the population, producing a serious shortage of labour, and so the opportunity for improved conditions. The government attempted to curb this by the Ordinance of Labourers of 1349, shown here, which was aimed at preventing workers from transferring from one master to another.

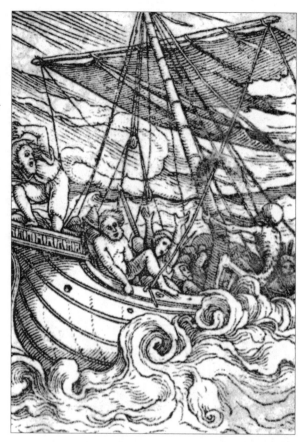

Right: 16 Plague was a disease spread along the trade routes and an added danger for sailors. Holbein shows a ship battered in a storm, with Death clinging to the broken mast.

Below: 17 London was a major seaport; Wyngaerde's view shows shipping on the Thames downstream from London, between the Tower and the royal palace of Greenwich in the distance.

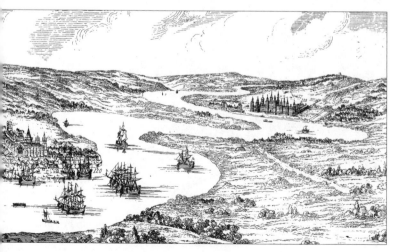

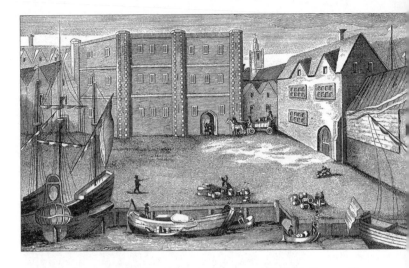

18 Customs dues on goods landed at London were paid at the Custom House, a short distance upstream from the Tower of London and close to the church of All Hallows by the Tower, seen to its right.

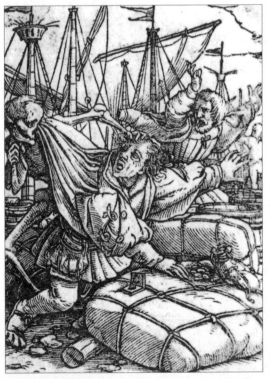

19 In Holbein's *Dance of Death* series, a merchant is eager to check his bales of newly landed goods, but Death is already plucking at his cloak. Textiles were regarded as one of the means by which plague was transmitted and the quarantining of shipping, which was introduced during the sixteenth century, required cargoes from suspect places of origin to be opened and aired.

Right: 20 Henry VIII was extremely fearful of plague and left London when an outbreak threatened to erupt. The first coherent measures to limit the spread of the disease were taken during his reign.

Below: 21 Following the destruction of the royal living quarters at Westminster Palace by fire in 1512, Bridewell Palace was adapted as the king's residence in London, although it was in a built-up part of the City. By 1660 it had become a prison.

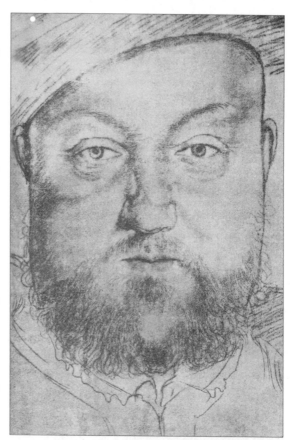

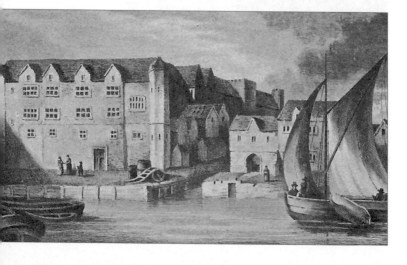

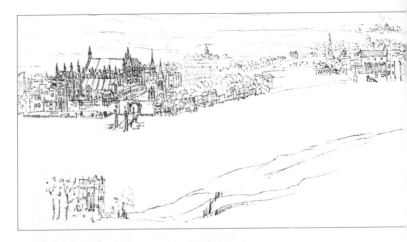

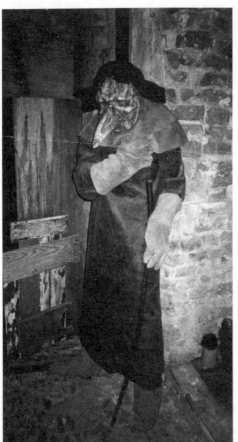

Above: 22 Henry VIII began the development of York Place as the royal palace of Whitehall, shown only sketchily by Wyngaerde, alongside the Thames between Westminster, with its abbey and St Stephen's church, and Durham House, close to the right of the drawing. St Martin's-in-the-Fields is behind Durham House, with St Giles-in-the-Fields beyond.

Left: 23 The plague doctor's costume consisted of a waxen robe, long gloves, boots, and a distinctive hood and mask, which had a bird-like beak filled with herbs, so that all of the skin was protected and the doctor breathed fragrant air.

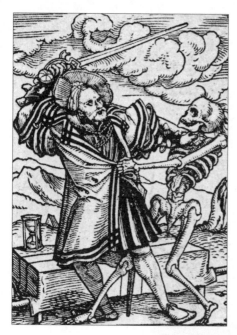

24 Despite precautions, including avoiding infected areas, plague still struck victims in all social groups. Holbein shows that a nobleman's weapons were futile, for Death pulls at him as his life, measured by the hourglass, is ebbing away and his coffin awaits.

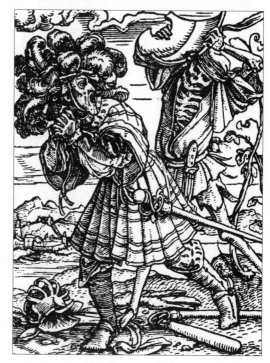

25 Holbein develops a similar theme in 'Death and the Count', as Death takes away the count's armour, leaving him defenceless.

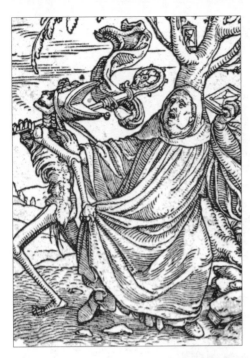

26 In a scene from the *Dance of Death*, an abbot is pulled away by the skeletal figure of Death masquerading as a bishop, with a mitre and crozier.

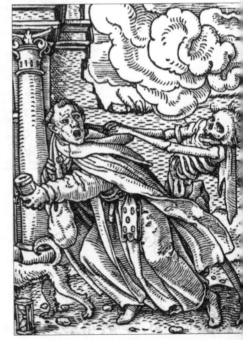

27 Even a poor friar, collecting alms and carrying his food, cannot escape Death, which pulls him back as he attempts to flee.

Right: 28 A nun, carrying her rosary, is taken from her convent by Death, to the horror of her fellow nun. The hourglass shows that her time has come. Nunneries and monasteries were no safe refuges during epidemics; in 1515 plague killed twenty-seven nuns of the Poor Clares at their house at the Minories.

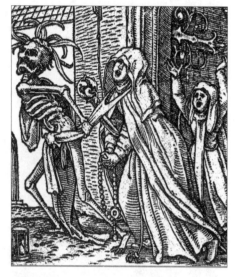

Below: 29 A section of the plan-view of London in Georg Braun and Frans Hogenberg's *Civitatis Orbis Terrarum* (1572), with St Paul's at the centre. Mid-Tudor London was increasingly wealthy and was growing rapidly, despite periodic plague epidemics, including a severe one in 1563.

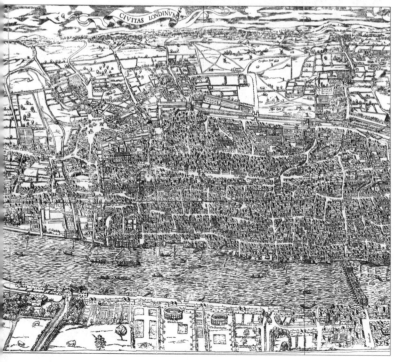

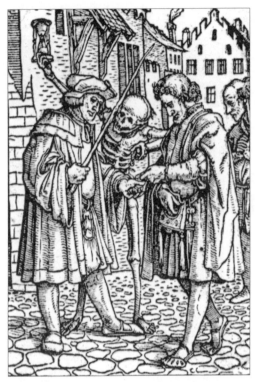

30 The leading citizens were responsible for enforcing the plague regulations. Holbein shows the town notables completing a transaction, but Death, with his hourglass, stands by listening to their conversation.

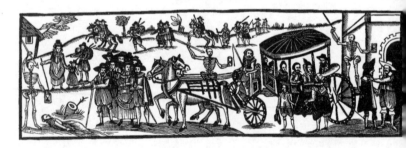

Above: 31 Many of those who could afford to leave fled from the city during an epidemic. In this woodcut from *A Looking-glasse for City and Countrey* (1630) they travel by coach, on horseback and on foot, yet Death, with spear and hourglass, stalks them, and has already claimed a victim.

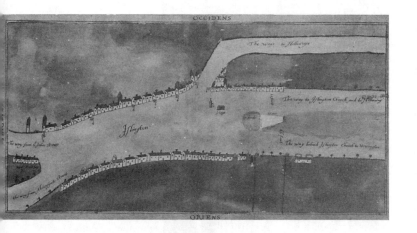

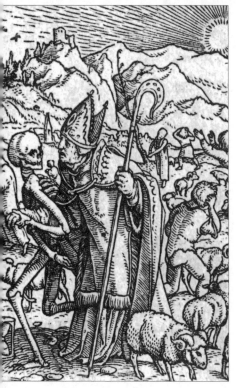

Above: 32 Some who fled from plague in London went to nearby villages, such as Islington, shown here on a mid-sixteenth-century plan.

Left: 33 Contemporaries debated whether the senior clergy should remain in the city during a plague outbreak, but Death leads this bishop away through the fields. The people are distraught as their spiritual shepherd is taken from them, while the sheep look on.

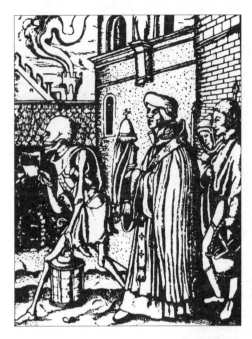

34 The parish clergy were expected to continue to serve their parishes, providing comfort, supervising the distribution of alms and conducting burial services. Plague burials were conducted at night, so Death carries a lantern.

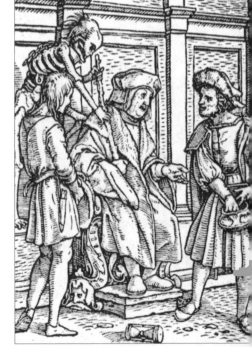

35 The magistrates oversaw the maintenance of law and order and the administration of the government's plague policies, but even as the judge is speaking, Death is reaching out for him.

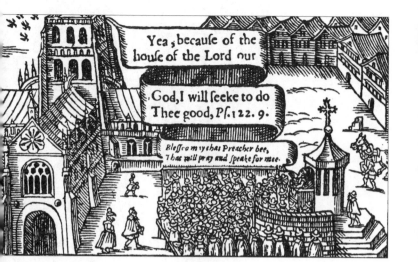

Yea, because of the house of the Lord our God, I will seeke to do Thee good, Pf. 122. 9.

Bleſſed my that Preacher bee, That will pray and ſpeake for mee.

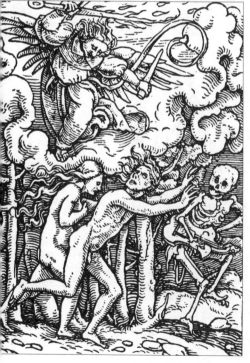

Above: 36 Sermons delivered from the pulpit at Paul's Cross in the cathedral churchyard attracted large congregations. Here Thomas White condemned plays as a cause of plague in a sermon in 1577. During plague outbreaks the authorities disapproved of such gatherings, but their orders were difficult to enforce, as Londoners continued to attend services.

Left: 37 Plague was widely regarded as a divine punishment, sent to chastise a sinful people. When Adam and Eve were expelled from the Garden of Eden, which was then guarded by a cherubim armed with a flaming sword, Death was waiting for them.

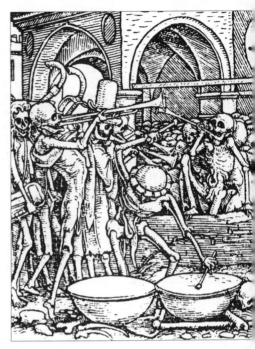

38 'The bones of all men': an image illustrating the universality of death. Skeletal figures make music; behind them is a churchyard packed full with the dead.

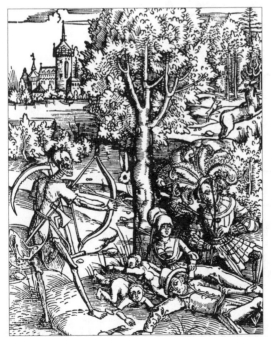

39 Those who tried to ignore the danger could not avoid sudden death. A stag has been shot with an arrow and a family enjoying a rest in an Arcadian landscape are themselves the target of the grim reaper's bow and arrow.

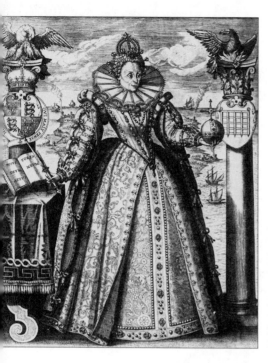

40 During the reign of Elizabeth I regulations were introduced to restrict the growth of London and those aimed to prevent the spread of plague were extended and codified, with a set of plague orders for London issued in 1583.

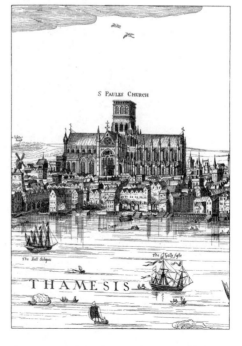

41 The churchyard of St Paul's was used by a number of parishes for burials, producing conditions that prompted the Lord Mayor to issue regulations in 1582 to restrict the numbers interred. This view of the cathedral is from Claes Visscher's *Panorama of London* of 1616.

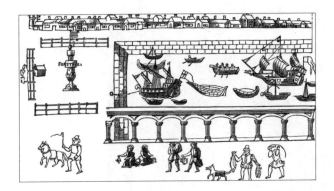

42 Billingsgate market, between London Bridge and the Tower, drawn by Hugh Alley in 1598. John Stow noted that the vessels that put in there unloaded grain, oranges, onions, and other fruit and root crops, as well as fresh fish. The measures aimed at preventing plague included the quarantining of ships from places suffering from an epidemic.

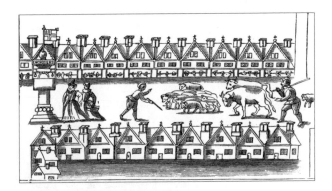

43 Alley's drawing of Eastcheap, one of the city's flesh markets. He shows the carcasses and joints of meat on poles in the butchers' shops, and livestock being driven along the street, but not the slaughter houses, the offal from which was regarded as a health risk.

arrangements had to be made so that they did not need to 'wander abroad and thereby infect others', but also recognised that some of those who were able to provide for themselves, and who were ordered to remain in their houses and avoid company, nevertheless 'very dangerously and disorderly misdemean themselves'. The justices were given the authority to levy a tax in their town or city and, if that proved inadequate, to apply to the county justices to extend it for five miles around, with powers to distrain goods in lieu of payment and to arrest those who refused to pay. With such arrangements for the necessary financial support in place, stricter enforcement of household quarantine could be applied, and the Act provided that those who had been instructed to stay in their houses but

> ...wilfully and contemptuously disobey such direction and appointment, offering and attempting to break out and go abroad, and to resist, or going abroad and resisting such keepers or watchmen as shall be appointed... to see them kept in; that then it shall be lawful for such watchmen with violence to inforce them to keep their houses; and if any hurt come by such inforcement to such disobedient persons, that then the said keepers, watchmen and any other their assistants, shall not be impeached therefore.

An infected person who defied the order to remain indoors and went into the company of others with an uncured plague sore was to be adjudged a felon and so be liable to the death penalty. These were harsh measures indeed, indicative of both the certainty of the government that household quarantine was the answer in restricting the spread of plague and the degree of exasperation felt by the authorities whose duty it was to enforce it. But by granting such powers and immunity to the parish officers who had to administer the quarantine, they were sowing the seeds of conflict and lasting resentment in the communities in which both the sick and the officers lived. And if, as was implicit in the Act, the disease was infectious, then a greater and more immediate danger to the officers than social ostracism was the physical contact necessary to restrain a plague victim who resisted incarceration. The very harshness of the Act made it unlikely that its provisions would be carried out in full, and so the problem remained unresolved.

Other aspects of plague control were not neglected. Attempts were made in 1602 to clear unauthorised and poor housing, but they were small-scale efforts which penalised an unlucky few and could not hope to stem the tide. Yet the orders against new buildings in London were reiterated in a proclamation of 1608, in which the evils of the city's growing population were declared to be 'dearth of Victuals, infection of Plague, and manifold disorders'. Filth, dunghills and 'stinking rubbish' spawned plague by contaminating the air. The authorities persevered with the enforcement of regulations aimed at improving the cleanliness of public places. In 1610, orders were issued aimed at cleaning up Westminster, with two scavengers appointed to carry away the human manure thrown into the streets, but the system did not work efficiently, for in 1613 the inhabitants of St Martin's Lane still threw their 'dust and Soyle in heaps before their Doores'.

Starchmaking was regarded as another source of miasmic air, through the foul smell that the process generated, as was made explicit in royal proclamations issued during these years. The monopoly on starchmaking was revoked in 1601 and the numbers who subsequently began to operate as starch-makers alarmed the government, both because of the amount of wheat that the industry consumed, which could raise the price of bread, and the health risk. A Starchmakers' Company of London was incorporated in 1607, but suspended in 1610 when starchmaking was forbidden, in a proclamation which declared that it 'may be one great cause to continue that dangerous Infection of the Plague, which hath (to our great griefe) bene generally dispersed amongst our people of late yeeres, by meanes of the same'. Not until 1622 was the Company reconstituted. Perhaps more effective were actions such as that taken by the churchwardens of St Margaret's, Westminster in 1610, when they paid for salt to 'destroy the fleas' in their pew. Certainly, the attempts to cleanse the air were not altogether successful, for while Dekker eulogised his native city as a 'Fownt, where milke and hony springs: Europs Jewell; Englands Jem', a contemporary, yearning for fresh air, condemned it as 'a great, vast, durtie, stinking cittie'.

The Privy Council continued to keep up the pressure on the corporation, by insisting that the regulations should be fully enforced. If the air and the weather were sound, then the citizens' own negligence must be to blame. In 1606, the Lord Mayor replied that the provost marshal went to the infected houses twice every day, accompanied by two of his own officers, to ensure that they were being guarded by the warders and that they had the printed notices upon their doors. Yet in the same year one of the bailiffs of Westminster displayed either an ignorance of the regulations or a reluctance to enforce them without higher authority, when he informed the Earl of Salisbury that he had shut up a partition door in a house where plague had been diagnosed, but asked if the street door was to be closed as well. Whatever the reason for his uncertainty, he had failed to grasp the principle that swiftness of action was required in such cases.

The king showed an interest in the measures which the Council adopted, comparing them with those issued in Scotland. In October 1609, the date of the queen's return to Whitehall was determined by the number of plague deaths in the Bill, and the absence of the court was seen as a way of coercing the citizens into closer observance of the regulations, in case it kept away longer and more often than before. Other towns could benefit from London's misfortune, as they were well aware. In 1605, the mayor and burgesses of Hertford had no compunction in pointing out that the plague was so bad in London that the Michaelmas Law term should not be held there, while in Hertford 'the courts as yett do stande readye buylte in the castell there for the same purpose'.

The question of the prohibition of public performances and closure of the playhouses during dangerous times was also dealt with. Anxieties about the numbers of people assembling at them may not have been misplaced. Those built as amphi-theatre playhouses, with open yards, such as the Globe and the Rose, could hold audiences as large as 3,000, while the hall playhouses, which were entirely under cover, had much smaller capacities, but even so had space for several hundred playgoers. Daily audiences in the early seventeenth century could have been as high as 5,000. A warrant of the Privy Council issued in April 1604 permitted the players to begin acting again after the epidemic, with the proviso that if the weekly number of plague deaths exceeded thirty, then 'they shall cease and forbear any further publicly to play'. Given the enlarged area covered by the Bills and the increase in population, this was a much stricter limitation than hitherto.

The weekly figures for 1604 and 1605 are incomplete, but those for 1606 and 1607 show that between early July and mid-November in both years plague deaths were higher than the specified number of thirty. An even longer closure of the playhouses was enforced between the last week of July 1608 and the first week of December 1609, when the number of plague deaths never fell below thirty. The players could tour provincial cities which were plague-free, when London was infected, which in epidemic years was from the early summer until at least December. But plague mortality in the capital did not always follow that pattern, and the criterion set by the Privy Council meant that there were no public performances for long periods during the early years of James' reign.

William Shakespeare's troupe was designated the King's Players by a patent issued by James soon after he arrived in London in 1603. He gave them £30 for their 'mayntenaunce and releife' during the epidemic in that year, which was a small sum compared to the £10 for each performance before the king or receipts from the playhouses when they were open. The Globe was closed for sixteen months in 1608–09 because of the plague, and the King's Players were granted £40 as 'rewarde for their private practice in time of infecction', with a further £30 in March 1610 for having been unable to perform publicly in London for six weeks, when they had acted before the court. During that Christmas season of 1609–10, the King's Players had acted thirteen plays for the court and other companies eleven. In April 1610, *Macbeth* and *Othello* were performed at the Globe, although the playhouses were closed later that summer, from 12 July to 15 November, and again for the week 22–29 November. When the number of plague deaths declined after 1610, they could be opened without restraint, but for only a part of the year, as the private performances in halls in the aristocratic and legal districts occupied the winter months, while public playing during Lent was normally forbidden.

Playwrights were one of the groups most seriously affected by the lingering presence of plague during those years, but it also provided them with topical references and plot devices. In John Fletcher's *The Tamer Tamed* (*c.*1603/4–1611), Petruchio feigns illness to arouse his wife's sympathy, but she counters his ploy by declaring the illness to be plague – she had seen the tokens on his body – so that the house is closed, with him quarantined inside it. Her apparent cruelty is tempered by her promise to keep him well supplied while he is incarcerated. Fletcher drew attention to the ease with which the quarantine system could be misused by someone with spiteful intentions, while Ben Jonson, in *The Alchemist* (1610), employed the context of a sealed house as the setting for dubious activities. The master has fled and closed the house, leaving one servant to look after it. Mocking the obsessive concern with the numbers of plague deaths recorded in the Bills of Mortality, Jonson gave the servant the line that the master could be relied on not to return to London 'While there dyes one, a weeke, O'the plague'. When he appears unexpectedly, the servant has to explain to his accomplices that he had meant one death a week within the walls, not within the liberties. Playgoers would have understood the distinction. The servant claims to have shut the house up for a month because of the plague, which, of course, would have deterred unwelcome attention from the swindling that had been practised in his master's absence. But he now declares that the victim had been a cat, who had been 'Convay'd away, i'the night' – an allusion to the practice of surreptitiously moving the dead and dying from houses in the City – and the servant had intended to burn rose-vinegar, treacle and tar to purify the air.

In *Romeo and Juliet*, Shakespeare used enforced household quarantine as the device whereby Friar John is unable to deliver the message to Romeo informing him that Juliet had taken a potion that had made her insensible, and she was not dead. The friar, suspected by the searchers of coming into contact with plague victims, is confined in a house and they 'Seal'd up the doors, and would not let us forth'. Without this information, Romeo assumes the worst and returns to Verona, and from that point the story moves on to its tragic climax. Shakespeare referred to another aspect of plague in *Timon of Athens*, in which he alluded to the connections between divine punishment for sinfulness, foul air and plague, with Timon telling Alcibiades, 'Be as a planetary plague, when Jove / Will o'er some high-vic'd city hang his poison / in the sick air'. More simply, in *Hamlet* he described the air as 'a foul and pestilent congregation of vapours'.

The immediacy of such scenarios receded after 1611, for plague deaths were recorded only in small numbers for the remainder of that decade and the early 1620s. Outbreaks elsewhere did not spread to south-east England. At Amsterdam, 1616, 1617, 1618, 1623 and 1624 were plague years, and an epidemic began in Bremen in 1623, but London was not affected. Indeed, in 1616 just nine plague burials were included in the Bills and in the following year the figure was only six, even though the disease had extended across the Low Countries. In response, an order was issued that bedding, feathers and other household goods could not be landed in the Thames, and in 1619, when plague was present in Rouen, two ships from there were held at Tilbury for twenty-five days.

Similar measures were taken regarding cargoes from other infected places, including Paris and other French towns in 1623. Only seventeen plague deaths were identified in London during that year, but vigilance was maintained, and because of plague in the Hague and elsewhere in the Low Countries, in August 1624 the Privy Council issued an order that care should be taken to prevent goods being imported from there which might carry the infection. On 1 October, the king prorogued Parliament because of 'a generall sicknesse and disease, which proves mortall to manie' that was prevalent in London and Westminster, with 400 burials during the previous week. This was a 'spotted ague', perhaps typhus fever, and not plague, for only eleven deaths were attributed to the disease throughout the whole of the year, and the prorogation was prompted less by disease than by the king's reluctance to face Parliament while the negotiations for the marriage of Prince Charles to the French princess Henrietta Maria were at a delicate stage.

In November, the negotiations with the French court were successfully concluded, and the marriage took place by proxy

on May Day 1625. James had died on 27 March and by the
time that his funeral was held on 7 May, the numbers dying
from plague were rising steadily. Even before the end of April,
the figure was causing concern: 'though it exceed not yet four
or five and twenty a week, yet the apprehension is more than
usual, and startles us very much, as well in regard of the time
of the year, and great concourse that of necessity must be, as
it is already dispersed in more than a dozen several parishes'.
By the middle of June, the weekly number had passed the
psychologically significant figure of 100. The parishes in the
north and east of the city were affected before the end of the
month and the disease then began to appear across the city.
The king and queen met at Dover on 13 June and entered
London, in the pouring rain, three days later. John Williams,
Bishop of Lincoln, was afraid for their safety and suggested
that they should travel by water rather than overland, to reduce
the number of contacts. Many families had left for the country and plague was appearing in different parts of the capital,
including Westminster, where a man had died of the disease
and the other six members of his family were being watched
anxiously in case they fell sick. The return for the last week of
the month showed 390 plague deaths and Charles' reign was to
begin with a major plague epidemic, as his father's had done.
Tentative plans for the coronation to be held in October had
to be abandoned, and it did not take place until 2 February
1626.

The disease, thought to have been transmitted from Holland,
was claiming victims in Great Yarmouth by February. The
Privy Council admonished the Lord Mayor and aldermen
and the justices of the adjoining counties to take adequate
steps to prevent plague spreading in London. They put the
usual measures in place, but the outbreak was not checked
and by early July 'no part of the City did stand free. Divers
fell down dead in the streets. All companies and places were

suspected which made all men willing to remove.' The Lord Mayor himself was absent for a few weeks while his house was closed after a plague case was diagnosed there, but the court remained and the king attended a service in Westminster Abbey on the Fast Day on 2 July. The fast was held to give thanks for the king's accession, to beseech God to cease the plague, and for the success of the fleet, which was due to set out to attack Cadiz. Prayers were offered at the same time for the end of 'the ceaseless rain which for a month past has fallen to the detriment of all kinds of crops'.

The weather fitted the pattern which contemporaries thought produced the plague; a hot and dry summer in 1624 was followed by a wet spring and early summer in 1625, with the rain continuing into July. But the spring was not a warm one, as in 1603. May and early June were unseasonably cool, but the number of plague cases continued to increase, giving rise to anxieties that the epidemic would worsen as it became warmer. In the middle of June, John Chamberlain commented: 'that which makes us the more afraid is, that the sickness increaseth so fast, when we have had for a month together the extremest cold weather ever I knew in this season. What are we then to look for when heats come on, and fruits grow ripe?' The physician Stephen Bradwell feared a 'deluge of destruction', and the rain and summer warmth did indeed produce the conditions which were conducive for the plague. The number of victims rose steadily during July, and at the end of the month it was pointed out that 'August is called the month of corruption, which is not yet come'.

The court moved away from Whitehall to Hampton Court on 4 July, but stayed for only a short time, as a case of plague was identified there. Many of the members of both Houses of Parliament had left already, but Sir Francis Nethersole, the member for Corfe Castle, stayed on, and in mid-July commented that the increase in plague deaths 'doth cause such a distraction and consternation in men's minds that the like was never seen in our age'. The anxious citizens were comparing the numbers in the Bills with those for the equivalent week in 1603, and when they rose to a much higher level they 'fled away as out of a house on fire'. Parliament was adjourned on 11 July, because of the poor attendance and the risk of the plague, to meet in Oxford on 1 August. Nethersole could then justify his departure; others had less excuse. Dekker believed that between the start of June and the middle of July, 4,000 houses had been closed, based on the number of printed papers issued, but that five times as many people had left London as had died. The city was 'almost desolate', because the rich had run away, leaving the poor 'in sorrow, in sicknesse, in penury, in unpitied disconsolations'.

The flight from London in 1625 provoked more righteous indignation than in any previous epidemic. This may have been because it was indeed larger than ever before. The number of baptisms in seven affluent City parishes for the plague months July to October shows a fall of just one per cent in 1563, compared with the number for the previous five years, but a drop of forty per cent in 1603 and of seventy per cent in 1625. This does not necessarily reflect the proportion of the total population of those parishes which had left, as pregnant women are more likely to have moved away than other groups, but it may be indicative of the scale of the evacuation in each of those plague years.

Dekker castigated the wealthy 'run-awaies' for abandoning the city 'in the midst of her sorrowes, in the height of her distresse, in the heavinesse of her lamentations'. Benjamin Spencer was no less censorious. In his *Vox Civitatis, or Londons Complaint against her Children in the Countrey*, he declared that the city had suffered economically by the flight of so many of its inhabitants, blaming the rich especially, for they had begun the process. When they had gone, 'then hath the middle sort little to doe; so that in fine, they will not finde themselves very needfull: and let them goe too and then others shall have nothing to doe', and when they had left, only the poor who had no escape into the country remained. With so many gone, the clergy and physicians felt that they did not need to stay, nor did the magistrates, who could appoint officers 'to keepe the poor folkes in order'. Spencer, a clergyman, objected to those who decided to leave, because in his opinion 'a Common-wealth is a body, and one member me thinkes should nourish another; but especially in a Christian Common-wealth'.

Those who had gone were uncharitable, taking their money with them and not paying their debts, nor making donations to help the poor. Admittedly, some had made such contribu-tions, 'but the most have not'. And they were also heartless in condemning the poor, as if God had chosen them for pun-ishment. The poor had indeed drawn His chastisement upon themselves by being 'for the most part, ill livers, intemperate of tongue, and appetite, grosse feeders, and such as disorderly thrust themselves into danger', which made them susceptible to other diseases as well as plague. But Spencer did recognise that plague 'takes hold on them more than others, because they be most in number', and believed that the disease did not strike at random, but took those 'appointed to die'. Yet he was inconsistent and, while he hoped that the city would be purged of 'vitious persons', he also recognised that 'Some good men are taken away', who could hardly be spared because 'heere is so few upon the earth'.

Spencer, like Clapham, questioned whether plague was infectious. It did not always infect the adjacent places, and he noted that the searchers, keepers, sextons and bearers were 'seldomest taken with it'. He also derided the idea that the air was particularly dangerous during an outbreak and so the city should be avoided. Everyone breathed the same air, and so did domesticated animals, and yet many escaped infection despite being exposed to the malodorous atmosphere. It would be more polluted after the epidemic, when everyone had returned and activity was again at its previous level, but the citizens would not leave for the country then.

The clergy had not entirely resolved the question of whether God sent the plague to remove the sinful from society, leaving the faithful unharmed, or whether it was indiscriminate in its choice of victims. But John Donne, Dean of St Paul's, shared Spencer's harsh view of some of the poor victims. In a sermon he asserted that those who had died in the epidemic included men who had been careless of their safety and had declared 'let us eat and drink, and take our pleasure, and make our profits, for tomorrow we shall die'. There were those who 'died in their sins, that sinned in their dying, that sought and hunted after death so sinfully, we have little comfort of such men'. They had made merry with eating and imbibing 'strong drink in riotous houses', had robbed houses and caught the plague from items they stole, or had visited brothels to try to catch syphilis, in the hope that it would give them immunity from plague. The outbreak had cleansed the city of people of that kind. Such an interpretation, that plague accomplished a selective cull of wrongdoers, could explain the unfortunate, perhaps even ill-omened, fact that the reigns of the first two kings of the dynasty had been ushered in with plague; for the epidemics of 1603 and 1625 could be regarded as purging the sins of the previous reigns. The alternative view, that they expressed God's disapproval of the new monarchs, was too uncomfortable to contemplate.

In any case, opinions such as Donne's were not wholly accepted. In *Balme from Gilead, to cure all diseases, especially the plague* (1626), Henry Roborough, the minister of St Leonard's Eastcheap, declared that those who apparently died before their time should not therefore be condemned as sinners. The numbers of children who died should have cautioned against the conclusion that the plague picked out wrongdoers and evil livers. Roborough's parishioner, Nehemiah Wallington, was well aware of the deaths of children and young mothers in the outbreak, noting in his journal gossip that 'threescore children died out of one alley' and, in another entry, that he had been told of 'threescore women with child and in childbed that died in one week in Shoreditch parish and scarce two that was sick with child that escaped death'. These exaggerated rumours had a basis in fact, for the deaths of children exceeded those of adults, as in previous epidemics. In the parish of St Dionis Backchurch, James Bostocke was buried on 17 August and four of his children also died before the end of the month, although his wife survived to remarry two years later. The father, two daughters and two sons of the Vidler family were buried at St Benet, Paul's Wharf during August, and the father, two sons and four daughters of the Wood family, at St Thomas the Apostle during September.

Donne was not an eyewitness of events in London during the epidemic, but spent the plague months at Chelsea, where he took the opportunity to correct and write out eighty of his sermons. Lady Ashburnham also retreated to Chelsea, as a guest of her kinswoman, the Duchess of Buckingham, where she prepared a devotional book of guidance for her daughters, published twenty years later as *A Ladies Legacie to her Daughters*. Daniel Featley, Rector of Lambeth and chaplain to the Archbishop of Canterbury, spent the time composing a book of instructions, hymns, and prayers, which, published in 1626 with the title *Ancilla Pietatis; or the hand-maid to private devotion*, became immensely popular and went through six editions by 1639.

Some who stayed in London, unable to leave, also passed their time profitably. William Lilly was one of two servants left behind when his master decamped to his native Leicestershire. With time on his hands, Lilly bought a bass viol and took

music lessons, played bowls with friends in Lincoln's Inn Fields
and went to funerals and other services, at his own church of
St Clement Danes and at St Antholin's, where a sermon was
delivered every morning. One day he passed only three people
on his way from his house at Strand Bridge to St Antholin's
in Budge Row. Admittedly this was at half-past six in the
morning, but he had to go roughly a mile and his direct route
would have taken him through a normally busy quarter of the
City, down Fleet Street, up Ludgate Hill, past St Paul's and
along Watling Street. Despite going out and about in the city,
he was 'nothing at any time visited, though my conversation
was daily with the infected'. He recalled that the minister of
St Clement Danes also escaped without any sickness, even
though he officiated at every funeral, whether the deceased
had died of the plague or not. Yet both of the clergymen who
assisted him at a service on a Sunday in August were taken
ill with plague that day; one died on the following Thursday
and the other took thirteen weeks to recover. Other clergymen stayed, including William Crashaw, rector of St Mary's,
Whitechapel, who buried as many as forty or sixty victims a
day, but survived the epidemic, dying in 1626.

Nehemiah Wallington and his household remained in St
Leonard's Eastcheap and the whole family kept in good health
through the worst of the outbreak, until October. Then, one
Saturday afternoon, a servant girl complained of 'a pricking
in her neck', a symptom of the plague. On the following
morning their daughter, not yet three years old, fell ill with
the disease and 'she continued in great agonies (which were
very grievous to us, the beholders) till Tuesday morning', when
she died. Nehemiah was beside himself with grief, although
his wife found it easier to accept the loss of their daughter's
life, saying that 'I do freely give it again unto God, as I did
receive it of him'. Surrounded by a numerous family who
lived close by, it may not have occurred to them to move

away, even if they had possessed the economic means to do so. Raphael Thorius, a physician and author of *Hymnus Tabaci* (1610), presumably could have left but chose to remain, and died at his house in London of the plague. John Fletcher, the dramatist, had the opportunity to leave, for he was invited to go into East Anglia to avoid the risk, but he 'stayd but to make himselfe a suite of Cloathes, and while it was making, fell sick of the Plague and dyed'. His tailor described to John Aubrey more than forty years later how, while treating his arm for an injury, he had 'found the Spotts upon him'. In Fletcher's case, vanity outweighed prudence, and he was buried in the parish of St Saviour's, in Southwark, when he could have been in the relative safety of East Anglia.

John Boston was clerk of that parish, having held the post since 1604. His duties included keeping the accounts and preparing the monthly bill of baptisms, marriages, churchings and burials. The number of burials rose sharply, from forty in February and forty-three in March to sixty-five in April, 101 in May, 180 in June, and 539 named persons 'and many unknowne' in July. It was the increase in deaths during July which prompted an exodus from the parish, for:

the Infeccon of the Sicknes and plague in July in the bill menconed increasinge and groweinge to such an height of extreamity and foarce the contagion whereof beinge lamentably spread almost through all the said parishe the danger was soe great that the minister of the said parishe withdrewe himself from doeinge his dutie and excersinge his function in celebratinge devyne service within the said parishe as usually before tyme hee had done and the then churchwardens and the nowe churchwardens or the most parte of them together with the rest of the most able parishioners in estate of the said parishe withdrewe themselves likewise from theire howses and habitacons into remote places and deserted the said John

Boston beinge a deacon to celebrate devyne service and per-
forme the Rites of Burrialls as they should happen within the
said parishe wch said Charge & Care the said John Boston was
enforced to undertake and was Constreyned to departe with
and leave... Sarah his wife and Twoe of his smalle children with
her and to his great greife to send them into the countrey from
him exposinge himself to unspeakable wattchinges labour and
travell [travail] both daie and night.

From the beginning of August until 15 September, there were
1,078 burials in the parish, hastening the departure of those
who could get away. Those who remained were chiefly 'the
poorer sorte', many of them so destitute that they did not
leave enough money to pay the burial fees. As many as thirty
or forty bodies a day were left at the burial ground during the
worst of the epidemic, without any indication of their identity.
This body dumping was done to avoid payment of the fees
and also, presumably, by relatives desperate not to have their
house closed. Boston had to try to discover who they were,
but was unable to collect fees for roughly a third of the burials.
The lists include his record of the interment of servants and
many poor people, such as the entry for 16 August noting the
burial of 'John Bassett, a boy, and divers other poore unknown'.
In September he was taken ill, but, conscientious to the last,
before he died he spoke out of an open window, so as not to
pass on the disease, to explain the financial position to Richard
Wright, a grocer. He also mentioned it to the two women who
nursed him, and survived. Boston was buried on 22 September,
as the epidemic began to wane, with 570 burials during the
month, but just ninety in October.

Boston's widow married Robert White and, although she
handed over money which she found in the house, the vestry
was not satisfied that all of the fees collected had been accounted
for, and sued Sarah and Robert for £62 8s in outstanding fees.

According to Richard Wright, testifying on behalf of the vestry, the description of a mass departure was exaggerated and 'Riche middle sorte and poore people' had all died in the parish during the outbreak. Two members of the vestry are indeed recorded among the burials in the register, but it is significant that the vestry, which normally met frequently, did not assemble at all between 28 June and 7 October, even though there were pressing matters to deal with. Wright's contention is not borne out by other evidence, and although St Saviour's did include unsavoury districts, containing brothels and alehouses, in other respects it was a stable and bustling area, not greatly different from the rest of the capital, where the absence of so many citizens had a marked effect. The case highlights conditions in a parish during such a severe epidemic, and the strains which they placed on parochial administration and a dedicated officer who remained to carry out his duties, which cost him his life.

Shortly after Parliament reconvened at Oxford, the House of Lords turned its attention to the effect of the plague on London. It requested that the king issue a charitable brief for collections throughout the country, as provided for by the Act of 1604, which was done on 11 August. The Lords also issued an order aimed at tackling the problems faced by the poor in London, Westminster, the out-parishes and Stepney, who 'in this time of the plague now reigning in those parts, are less subject to good orders, being left destitute of convenient relief, in respect that the rich and able citizens, and other inhabitants of all sorts, being departed thence for avoiding the infection, have not taken sufficient order for relief of the poor people remaining behind'. All those who qualified to pay tax were to pay a double levy during the epidemic, or more if the magistrates thought it necessary. Aware that the collections could be delayed because 'very many are removed from London', the City chamber, or its Bridgehouse estate, was authorised to lend £1,000 until the funds were received. This was reimbursed out of the receipts from collections authorised by the charitable brief. Those who refused to pay could be referred to the House of Lords itself, which undertook 'to punish them so exemplarily as shall be a terror unto others'. Finally, the Lords commended the action of those livery companies which had cancelled their celebratory dinners and donated the money which would have been spent on them to the fund for poor relief. The City itself was able to raise enough money to make provision for its poor, and so did not need to draw from the charitable receipts that were collected.

This did not apply across the whole of the capital. The Duke of Buckingham took an active role in Parliament's involvement with the problem of providing relief, and described the poor as being 'in a miserable case' because of the plague and 'want of commerce'. The impact was described in a letter sent from London on 1 September: 'The want and misery is the greatest here that ever any man living knew: no trading at all; the rich all gone; housekeepers and apprentices of manual trades begging in the streets, and that in such a lamentable manner as will make the strongest heart to yearn'. The near-collapse of normal business was highlighted by Dekker: 'If one Shop be open, sixteene in a row stand shut up together, and those that are open, were as good to be shut; for they take no Money'. Only apothecaries, butchers, cooks and coffin-makers were thriving. Few people were walking in the streets and some houses had nobody living in them. John Taylor also conveyed the emptiness of London:

> Houses shut up, some dying, some dead,
> Some (all amazed) flying, and some fled.
> Streets thinly man'd with wretches every day,
> Which have no power to flee, or meanes to stay,
> In some whole street (perhaps) a Shop or twaine
> Stands open, for small takings, and less gaine

Food was in short supply, because the country people were not bringing their produce into the city in the usual quantities. Spencer commented that London could 'scarce get provision from the Countrey' and that those who remained were driven 'almost beyond their abilities to find them necessaries'.

Resentment of the country people was increased by their hostile reaction to refugees from London who were looking for somewhere to stay. As Taylor recognised, this antagonism was based on a dread of the plague:

The name of London now both farre and neere,
Strikes all the Townes and villages with feare;
And to be thought a Londoner is worse,
Than one that breakes a house, or takes a purse.

Henry Petowe expressed indignation that Londoners were being treated so badly by those with whom they had regular contact, as suppliers of food. If refugees from London so much as attempted to pass through a village, they were told 'No, for you are Londoners' and were kept out by countrymen wielding 'Pichforks, Staves, Hookes, browne Bills, and such like rustick Weapons'. John Evelyn was four years old when the epidemic began and he was sent to live with his grandfather in Lewes, later recalling that 'I well remember the strict Watches, and examinations upon the Ways as we pass'd'. A woman with plague symptoms nevertheless managed to reach Hereford, where the churchwardens of All Saints parish ordered that she should be sent back to London; protection of the community took precedence over charity and pity. Most towns would not admit travellers who did not have a health certificate. A man from London died in the fields outside Southampton, but fear of the disease was overridden by greed, because he 'had good store of money about him, which was taken before he was cold'. John Donne thought that some were carrying enough money

to have bought the village where they died, and heard of one
man who had £1,400 on his person when he expired.

John Gore, the Lord Mayor, complained about the order of
the Essex justices that carriers who had gone to London should
then stay within their houses for fourteen days, pointing out
that if those remaining in the city became short of food there
could be disorders, which the few remaining magistrates would
be unable to control. The Council, fearful of unrest, directed
the Essex justices to withdraw their order and commanded
that designated marketplaces should be established around the
city, in Mile End Green and Woods Close to the east, Tothill
Fields and St James' Fields to the west, and St George's Fields
on the south side of the river. In any case, preventing trade with
London was economically damaging, and in mid-September
the Deputy Lieutenants of Essex reported to the Privy Council
that the clothiers, graziers, market gardeners and hop-growers
could not sell their produce because of the plague in London,
and that the situation had been exacerbated by a deficient
harvest, caused by the wet summer. In fact, across England and
Wales agricultural price levels in 1625 were only nine per cent
above the average for the preceding five years, although this
figure probably conceals higher prices locally due to shortages
during the plague months.

Attempts to modify established patterns of trade to overcome the effects of the epidemic could be futile. The Council
proposed to move the staple for cloth sales from London to
Reading, enabling the West Country clothiers to sell their
stock and so continue with production. If they had to reduce
output, problems would arise with the increasing pressure on
poor relief and possible unrest in the clothing districts. Reading
could provide storage facilities and had communication along
the Thames; the merchants would not be afraid to go there and,
importantly, foreign buyers could be confident that the cloth
had not come from an infected place. They would not trade in

London because of the epidemic, 'which by experience wee finde to cause our shipping in many places to bee rejected'.

The Council then discovered how difficult policy-making could be during an epidemic, because the members of the Merchant Adventurers Company were scattered and the company did not respond to the proposal, in writing or in person. The only reaction from one of its members came in a letter sent by William Towerson, in Essex, protesting that the action was unnecessary because less cloth was made during harvest time, when labour was employed in agriculture, and by the time that cloth output rose again later in the year the plague would have lessened. He also believed that the merchants would not go elsewhere to buy. The Wiltshire clothiers also declared that the trade should continue as before, and they won an important concession when the Council allowed them to continue to sell their cloth in London, specifying only that it must be done by private contract, not in an open market, and the cloth should be taken to the merchants' warehouses without risk of spreading the disease.

The Council's compromise acknowledged London's primacy in the marketing of cloth and it was influenced, too, by the severe recession which had beset the cloth-making areas in the early 1620s. The effects had been so serious that a commission had been set up in 1622 to report on the causes of the slump in the trade and submit recommendations for its revival. The plague struck as the industry was beginning to recover, and the Council was so anxious to limit its impact as far as possible that it was prepared to be adaptable. Even so, the quantity of cloth brought to London for sale in 1625 was down by twenty per cent on the average figure for the previous five years.

The economic impact of the epidemic was such that, as in the first year of James' reign, the government's revenues were seriously reduced. Sir John Wolstenholme calculated the

loss to those who farmed the customs at £5,041 over the
year. The other taxes could be collected only with difficulty,
while the wealthier, tax-paying citizens were widely scattered,
and plague made the city a hazardous place for the collec-
tors, but the cost of James' funeral and the other expenses of
the new reign absorbed the reserves. By July the coffers were
'exhausted', with no money in the treasury, and the court's
needs were becoming desperate. Yet the king was determined
to fit out the fleet for a summer campaign against Spain.

Parliament granted him two subsidies, which would produce about £160,000, but when it reassembled at Oxford
the Crown claimed that £800,000 was required, and resorted
to demands for loans, issued under the Privy Seal, which
generated squeals of protest from those impoverished by the
epidemic. Indeed, this was not a good time to be asking for
more, with business so badly disrupted. The reaction in Surrey
and Middlesex was surprise and displeasure that loans should
be demanded while the two subsidies were being collected,
and as though economic conditions had not been affected by
the plague. Gideon Delaune, one of London's most prominent
apothecaries, complained that profits from his shop had fallen
because of the deaths of his servants, and Sir Robert Pye,
auditor of the Exchequer of Receipt, was warned that, because
of the plague, money could not be collected from those who
had it. The effects of the epidemic and the Crown's failure to
adapt to them undoubtedly contributed to the difficult relations between the king and his first Parliament.

The government's difficulties with financial matters were
similar to its problems supervising the regulations concerning
the plague. In both cases, practical enforcement was beyond its
control, but it became anxious because widespread refusal to
comply with the plague orders would bring authority generally into contempt. When the king came to Richmond Palace
towards the end of July, Londoners went there, in clear defiance

of the proclamation that no one from infected places should go near to any of the royal houses, and it was suspected that they were disguising themselves as countrymen so that they could follow the court. In October, the Council complained that they had received information that in Westminster 'those who have the sore running upon them goe as freely abroade conversing promiscuously with others as if they were not infected'. The justices were at fault in permitting this, especially as it was being done so close to Whitehall Palace. They were either negligent, to permit such a breach of the orders, or were absent as, the Councillors had to admit, they were themselves, being 'forced to disperse ourselves more than at any other time hath beene usuall'. But they urged the Lord Mayor and justices to remain during the crisis. The Council's instructions were based upon such information as they could receive from the city, although communication was a problem, and those struggling to deal with the crisis in London were bound to vindicate their own efforts in response to the Council's censures.

Some of the Council's orders were based on the experience of previous outbreaks, such as one to prevent vagrants from burgling empty houses, 'a thing practized as wee heare by dissolute and desperate persons in tymes of former contagion and plague'. Others were modifications of earlier policies. While Elizabeth's Council had attached importance to the efficacy of collective worship during an epidemic, this was now thought to be outweighed by the dangers of people gathering together and spreading the disease. The weekly fast was not to be observed in the churches of those parishes which were infected, but the parishioners were to pray in their own houses. And the churchwardens of the parishes free from plague were not to admit those from infected parishes to their services. Effectively, this meant that all Londoners who remained in the city could not attend the fast services, because plague had spread across the whole metropolis. St John Zachary near Aldersgate was the only one of the 122 parishes included in the Bills that did not record a death from plague during the year.

In practice, the citizens continued to go to church and to attend funerals, as in 1603. At the Dutch church, services were continued on Sundays and weekdays, and the response to the concerns of some members of the community that people with plague sores were attending church was to request them not to come to services or, if they wished to do so, to keep away from the worshippers, in a separate part of the church. This tolerant and sympathetic attitude disregarded the orders of the Council on both church services and household quarantine. A more brazen defiance of the Council's policies came on 24 September, when the full-scale funeral of Richard Robins, a captain of the Trained Bands, was celebrated at St Margaret, New Fish Street, attended by 240 citizen-soldiers and watched by a crowd estimated to have been as large as 10,000. After the service, the funeral procession passed through the streets to the Lord Mayor's house, where he generously distributed wine and claret among the mourners. This demonstrated that the city was not, in fact, virtually depopulated, but it also ignored the plague orders and may have been one of the reasons for the Council to lambast the Lord Mayor and aldermen a few weeks later, with the complaint that 'there hath beene greater slacknesse and neglect than may anie way stande with that care which you ought to have of your owne safety and welfare and the contentment of his Majesty'.

Awareness of the far greater scale of mortality in 1625 may have been a reason for the Council's complaint that the regulations had been neglected. But in the early stages of the outbreak the specified practices had been observed. On 24 April, the vestry of St Margaret Lothbury reacted to the death of a child of William Miller's from plague by ordering that the designated measures should be put in place, and closing the house, with its eight occupants. A week later,

Miller appealed for help and was lent £3 by the parish, to be repaid when he had recovered, but on 9 May he asked for more, 'which was very strange to the whole parish, having spent so much money in so shorte a time'. The vestry then asked Miller if he and the rest of his household were willing to go to the pesthouse (but did not order them), and he agreed. No doubt the vestry was relieved, even though it would have to pay more than £11 for the month they were kept there. Despite the cost, the arrangement was preferable to household quarantine because it relieved the vestry of the responsibility of supplying the household with provisions and of guarding the house, which was proving difficult: 'for many did venter & hasard themselves both strangers & others to see them', putting the neighbourhood at risk from the spreading of the disease.

As the epidemic worsened, the pesthouses became inadequate to accommodate the numbers who ideally should have been isolated in them, and the problem of restraining those who ought to be incarcerated in their houses, which had arisen in earlier outbreaks, recurred. By the end of August, the Privy Council admitted that the policy of separating the sick and their contacts from the rest of the population had broken down. Everyone who had been in the city could see for themselves that 'the whole and the sicke are suffered in all partes of the cittie promiscuously to converse together without any restrainte at all'. To increase the accommodation for the infected, the Council ordered that groups of small tents and cabins should be erected around the city, using 'a few boards and such materialles as may bee soone putt together', and well spaced. Those who were suspected to be suffering from plague were to be taken there at once, while the remaining members of the household were to serve their quarantine in the house. If the sick recovered, they were to be sent home after a month and the cabin and their clothes burned, with new ones built as long as they were required. Edinburgh had adopted this practice in 1585, and it was a refined version of the requirement of 1602 that plague suspects who had landed in England serve their quarantine in the fields. It addressed one criticism of the existing arrangements by separating the infected from the contacts, a practice widely adopted in the Italian cities. But it conflicted with the notion that plague sufferers going along the streets would spread the infection. And the Council may not have realised the irony of ordering the erection of shanty villages on the edge of the city, when its own policy was to remove all such shoddy buildings, many of which started life as temporary structures.

By the time that the Council changed its policy, the death toll was beginning to fall, if only because 'when the fuel lessens, the fire cannot be so great'. From 942 burials in the last week of June, the number rose steadily to 3,583 four weeks later. Between the last week of July and the second week of September, the weekly return recorded more than 3,000 burials, and the week of Captain Robins' funeral saw almost 2,000 burials. The high point of the epidemic across the city was the week ending 18 August, the week of the 'great bill', which recorded 5,205 burials, and for six weeks the numbers exceeded the highest weekly figure registered in 1603. The numbers fell steadily thereafter, and in the first week of October 833 burials were recorded, the lowest number for sixteen weeks. The total for the year was 54,265 burials. Of these, 35,417 were designated as plague, but doubts were expressed that the numbers returned as plague deaths were accurate. The reaction to the Bill for the first week in July was that 'by common opinion there died many more', and at the end of the month one observer thought that almost 1,000 of the 1,112 deaths registered as from other diseases in the previous week were in reality caused by plague, and those he sarcastically described as being from 'the invisible plague'.

As in 1603, the epidemic killed roughly twenty per cent of London's population. From the numbers of burials and baptisms for the two years, John Graunt concluded that 1625 was no more destructive of life than 1603 had been, allowing for the growth of the city, although there was a slight difference, with eight burials for every baptism in 1603 and 7.8 in 1625. The increase in the number of burials compared with the preceding years, in a sample of City and suburban parishes, shows that in eleven parishes the multiple in 1625 was lower than in 1603 and in three it was higher. Such computations are indicative, but the patterns of population were distorted during an epidemic. In the City parishes, the figure for the multiple of burials over the normal level was relatively low because of the numbers who had left. The highest ratios were for the parishes in the north-east and those south of the river, where the recorded deaths rose more than sixfold. While the proportion of the population which died in 1625 may have been slightly lower than in 1603, the number who died was much higher than in any previous year, and the outbreak in 1625 became known as the last great plague.

These two major epidemics had erupted despite the coherent measures that had been put in place to prevent plague reaching England and to contain it when an outbreak began. In addition to the oversight of the Privy Council and the implementation of its policies by the Lord Mayor, aldermen and justices of the peace, acting through the local officers, Parliament had intervened to ensure financial support for the poor who needed assistance when quarantined. Even when this was tackled, the plague orders were neglected, disobeyed, or even challenged. The Council's conviction that the disease was contagious, and its spread could therefore be checked by isolating the victims, was not wholly accepted, either by those who were convinced that God sent and halted the plague or by the Londoners who, from their own experience, doubted whether the disease was indeed contagious. Without widespread support, the execution of the plague policies was difficult. They could not be implemented effectively by force, only by the acceptance and compliance of the citizens. But as no alternative strategy was available, the government's approach was to insist on the enforcement of the procedures, even though they had been seen to fail twice within a generation.

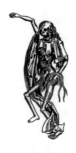

4

The Plague on the Wane?

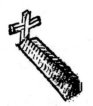

The epidemic of 1625 came in the early stages of a period of widespread outbreaks of plague across much of Europe. Some of these were related to military activity, especially the Thirty Years War, which had begun in Bohemia in 1618 and gradually spread to engulf much of central Europe, and the war between the United Provinces and Spain, which was suspended by a truce in 1609 but renewed in 1621. The early 1620s certainly saw a sharp increase in the number of places affected by plague and the figure remained high until the late 1640s. This coincided with a concentrated period of fighting, with the main theatres of the war, in Germany and the Low Countries, extended from time to time

by the shorter conflicts which erupted during this period of
diplomatic instability. In 1648, a general peace was concluded
which ended both the Thirty Years War and Spain's struggle
with the United Provinces, and the danger then diminished
somewhat, but did not disappear.

Between 1622 and 1646, France suffered the worst outbreaks
of plague in its history, including an epidemic in 1628–32
which claimed 750,000 victims. The disease spread into Italy
in 1629, during the early stages of the War of the Mantuan
Succession between France and Spain. A French army crossed
the Alps and, to support the Spanish effort, troops arrived in
Lombardy from Germany, where there had been an epidemic
in the previous few years, which had killed over half of the citizens of Augsburg in 1627 and 1628. The arrival of the armies
and those who moved with them, the 'camp followers', were
blamed for sparking the outbreak in Italy, known as the *peste di
Milano*. They certainly did not deign to observe the regulations
designed to limit the spread of disease and from Lombardy the
plague was dispersed across northern and central Italy, with
devastating effect. When it reached Venice, 46,490 died in the
city, perhaps a third of its inhabitants, while in Milan itself
60,000 of the city's population of 130,000 fell victim to the
disease.

England's direct military involvement was limited to a futile
expedition under the Protestant commander Count Ernst von
Mansfeld to recover the Palatinate for the king's son-in-law,
the Elector Palatine, in 1625, a raid on Cadiz later that year
and the occupation of the Île de Ré in 1627, to support the
Huguenots in La Rochelle. Charles followed a pacific foreign policy after the murder of the Duke of Buckingham in
1628, but London was at risk nonetheless, from its overseas
trade and the movement of soldiers and suppliers, especially to
and from the campaigns in the Low Countries and Germany.
Professional soldiers and gentlemen volunteers served with the

Dutch, Danish, Swedish, French, Spanish and Imperial armies, especially during the 1630s, when the king's policies were successful in avoiding conflict. War provided an honourable career and the opportunity to acquire wealth. At least 20,000 Britons served abroad between his accession and the outbreak of the Civil War in 1642 and there was an average of 4,000 with the Spanish army of Flanders during the 1630s. London was both a recruiting ground and the port of arrival for many of those returning from campaign, and remained by far the most important outlet for goods shipped abroad, which continued to increase, despite the decline in cloth exports.

At Amsterdam, 1626, 1629 and 1636 were plague years; Rotterdam suffered epidemics in those years and also in 1634, 1635 and 1637; and the outbreak which began at Bremen in 1623 continued intermittently until 1628. And so the policy of quarantining shipping had to be maintained and diligently executed. In 1629, the Privy Council warned the Lord Mayor that because of plague in and around Amsterdam, in the towns along the coasts of Brittany and at La Rochelle, he should ensure that no passengers or goods from those places were landed at London, and that nobody went aboard incoming vessels until it could be ascertained that plague was not present in the ports from which they had come. Goods were to be aired until they were thought to be free from the possibility that they harboured plague.

Other aspects of plague policy were reconsidered in the aftermath of the 'great plague' of 1625, with attention given to the effects of the outbreak and the lessons which could be learned. One result of the numbers of burials and the speed with which they were carried out was that during a storm in 1626 coffins buried too close to the surface were uncovered. The problem had been anticipated in the previous August, when the Council instructed the bishop of London to ensure that burials had at least three feet of earth over them, which was not being done. This provided an unpleasant reminder of the epidemic, and some chose to interpret the 'whirling and ghoulish' tempest as 'a sign against the Duke of Buckingham'. More seriously, the broken tombs were regarded as a hazard, from the corrupted air that emanated from them, although in the City parishes, at least, the majority of corpses had been buried in coffins. The register for St Dionis Backchurch notes that just nine of the ninety-nine burials there in 1625 were 'uncoffined'.

Parliament's reaction to the outbreak was prompted by Dudley Carleton in the House of Commons, who proposed the setting up of a Select Committee to draft a Bill 'to prevent Contagion', stipulating regulations based on those in force in such cities as Paris and Venice. The measures taken in London were evidently thought to be less stringent than those imposed by some continental cities, especially the Italian ones, which were admired, although they were no more successful in preventing periodic epidemics. But other business took precedence and the growing tensions between the Crown and Parliament prevented further consideration of the matter before the king resolved, in 1629, to rule without a Parliament. In any case, the problem came to seem less urgent, for the pattern of recurring outbreaks for a number of years, which had happened after the epidemic of 1603, was not repeated. The Bills of Mortality recorded 134 plague burials in 1626, just four in 1627, three in 1628 and none at all in 1629.

Although absent from London in 1629, plague was present elsewhere, notably in Cambridge, where the college authorities gave permission for the fellows and scholars to leave. In March 1630, the disease was recorded again in London, in St Giles-in-the-Fields, Shoreditch and Whitechapel, and the Council acted swiftly, ordering the reprinting of the plague orders, the choice of a building by the Middlesex justices to serve as a pesthouse and the closure of infected houses in the

City, with their occupants taken to the pesthouse. In April, it instructed the Lord Mayor to ensure that all of the infected houses were closed, marked with a red cross and the notice 'Lord have mercy upon us' set upon the doors, and that they should be guarded. The playhouses were shut and all public entertainments prohibited, as well as meetings at taverns and in the halls of the livery companies. Yet the numbers of plague deaths returned by the parish clerks were comparatively few, no more than single figures for most weeks during the spring, although they exceeded forty in July. The alarm probably was caused by the extent of the disease in the outer suburbs and the villages around London, and the fear that it would spread from Cambridge, which was suffering another serious epidemic.

Apprehensive of what might develop, Thomas Dekker was prompted to write another plague pamphlet, *London Looke Backe*, recalling 1625 and drawing lessons from that 'Yeare of Yeares', although written 'not to Terrifie, But to Comfort'. Using the analogy of a military engagement, he warned that so far 'the cannon of the Pestilence does not yet discharge, but the small shot playes night and day upon the suburbes'. Arrows were flying overhead and hitting some targets, and so he cautioned his readers to protect themselves. But what could be done? The answer was clear: reformation of conduct was required, because 'Repentance is a Silver Bell, and soundes sweetly in the Eare of Heaven'. The dire experience of the outbreak of 1625 should have brought such repentance and, in its turn, an alteration in behaviour. But that had not happened; the warning had not been heeded and the citizens remained sinfully defiant. Some who had recovered from the sickness had returned to their old ways and their conduct had even deteriorated; they had been drunkards before their sickness and 'were ten times worse, after they were well'. Dekker's interpretation of their behaviour at such a stressful time was a strictly moral one. He also judged harshly those who gathered roots and herbs to make medicines, assuring the victims 'stricken with Carbuncles, Blaynes, and Blisters' that they would cure them. Indeed, he thought that no help could be obtained from the authorised members of the medical professions either, for 'What Physitians, Doctors, Surgeons, or Apothecaries, have wee to defend us in so dreadfull a Warre? None, not any.'

Others hinted that the sins which may have helped to provoke God's wrath included the revival of Catholic practices in worship. Puritan ministers such as William Gouge were alarmed at the rise of Arminianism within the English Church and the presence of Roman Catholics in the queen's household, especially the twelve Capuchin friars who had recently been installed there. The writer of a private letter suggested that the outbreak of plague had given the king himself pause for thought and that he had forbidden anyone from attending mass, except the queen's servants. Outwardly, Charles was delighted at the birth of a son, the future Charles II, on 29 May; he attended a service of thanksgiving at St Paul's and gave the City £100 to help the plague victims. He decreed that the funds for poor relief were to be further augmented by contributions from the members of the livery companies, who were enjoined to donate half of the money that would have been spent on their feasts, which were cancelled. This was accompanied by the veiled threat that the king would 'take notice' of those who did not make such a contribution.

The Privy Council, which did not share Dekker's scepticism of the medical profession, asked the College of Physicians for a revised 'Advice', which accompanied the plague orders. One of the College's Censors was William Harvey, who reacted crossly by complaining that he and his colleagues had been ignored during the epidemic in 1625. But it responded quickly, nevertheless, and produced a new 'Advice', recommending prescriptions and good practices, such as the quarantining of the sick.

As the epidemic developed, the Council again belaboured the corporation and justices for not rigidly implementing the measures which should have been taken, and choosing as searchers unsuitable people, some of whom 'abuse the trust reposed in them, by concealeing the Infeccion'. Infected houses were not being closed quickly enough and the distinguishing marks were not being fixed to them, nor were they being watched properly, and those who guarded them were not being adequately supervised. Furthermore, the parishes were 'not affording sufficient mayntenance to such persons infected as are of the poorer sorte soe shutt upp, whereby they are necessitated to come abroade for releefe'. A part of the problem, it suggested, was that the justices were not taking 'so strict an account' of the 'subordinate Ministers and officers' as they should have done. Yet the parish officers at St Mary Zachary seem to have carried out their duties as prescribed, in sealing the house of Richard Stanton and his family, supplying them with provisions, appointing a warder to guard the house and paying for the burials of the two children who died of plague.

The outbreak did not prove to be as severe as the Council feared when, in November, it ordered that 10,000 quarters of corn should be shipped to London from Ireland because it was afraid of a food shortage and therefore an increase in plague in the city, 'which is the ordinary effect thereof'. Malnutrition was thought to be a contributory cause of plague, which helped to explain why those in the poorer districts suffered most. The epidemic of 1625 had indeed coincided with wet weather and a bad harvest and that had coloured the Council's thinking, but the pattern had not occurred in 1603, nor was it to do so in 1630. No week saw as many as eighty plague deaths recorded in the Bills and there were 1,317 deaths from the disease during the year, only 190 of them within the walls.

The plague had begun, but had been contained, which seemed to justify the government's policies and the effectiveness of their implementation. Letters from the Lord Mayor to the Council stressed that the searchers had carried out their duties honestly, that infected houses had been closed, marked and watched, and that funerals had been held at night and attended only by 'very few or none'. The Council appeared to acknowledge this success when it wrote to the Lord Mayor at the end of January 1631, commenting that the number of plague victims was 'so diminished as it was almost not considerable in so great a Cittie', before ordering continued strict attention to its edicts. The danger had not entirely passed and there was an increase in the numbers in the weekly Bill early in January, which was explained with the comment that the weather had been 'extraordinarilie warme for winter'. In the middle of March, the plague was said to have 'lingred and hunge aboute the skirts of this Citty all this last winter'.

Perhaps because of its continued presence, in March the Council wrote again to the College requesting advice, and it delegated consideration of the College's response to a committee, together with recommendations which had been received from the king's physician, Sir Theodore de Mayerne. The College's 'Advice' provided the prescriptions for preventatives and cures, and went much further in enumerating the 'Annoyances' which contributed to outbreaks of plague. Its authors made a connection between disease and the poor urban environment, caused by the increasing number of buildings and the lodging of inmates, which brought overcrowding and unhealthy conditions. Dirty streets and stagnant water created dangers if ditches and sewers were not cleaned out and ponds were allowed at inns. Those who died of plague should not be buried in churches and churchyards, too many burials were permitted in churches, and ducts from burials vaults and privies allowed foul air to seep out into the atmosphere. Air pollution was also caused by slaughterhouses and laystalls of manure, which were being created too near the city, while rotten fish, diseased cattle and musty corn, sold in public markets and even baked into bread, also contributed to the risks.

Mayerne's submission recommended the creation of a board of health along continental lines. This was to consist of twelve members, including the Lord Mayor, two aldermen, the Recorder, the bishop of London, members of the Privy Council and three members of the College of Physicians, one of whom 'hath beene a Traveller' and so had experience of how such a system was operated elsewhere. The board would have a fund for all expenditure that related to public health, including the employment of food inspectors, with powers to confiscate unwholesome meat, corn, beer and wine.

The measures concerning plague which he recommended were divided into those taken before an outbreak and those taken during an epidemic. It could be prevented by good intelligence of its presence on the continent, especially in the Low Countries, which Mayerne thought was the commonest source from which the disease was brought into England. Those coming from an infected area should be required to produce health certificates, as in Italy, and be subject to a forty-day quarantine in 'commodious houses' provided for the purpose. But poor strangers should not be allowed to land at the ports at all, because their dirtiness was a risk in itself. He regarded famine as a cause of plague and thought that the government should regulate food supplies, a policy which the Council had implemented during the previous autumn. In London, household quarantine should last for forty days, but ideally the sick ought to be separated from the healthy, and the relatives and contacts of those who were infected should also serve the period of quarantine. If implemented, this would have ended the practice, which was so resented by the citizens, of incarcerating together those with plague and those who were free from the disease, but suspected of being contacts.

Mayerne also recommended that London be split into five divisions for health purposes, each with its medical staff, including doctors, surgeons, apothecaries and women search-ers. Four or five pesthouses were required, one in Southwark and the others north of the Thames, with a principal hospital to be built at Chelsea or Paddington. This was to be known as Godshouse or the King's Hospital; Mayerne's inspiration was the L'Hôpital St Louis at Paris, erected by Henri IV between 1607 and 1612. The Council sent the corporation a memoran-dum describing the building, which clearly was intended to serve as the exemplar for the City's own project.

His concerns regarding the urban environment were similar to those expressed by the College: rubbish should be dumped in the streets only just before collection, ditches must be scoured, smelly trades and fish markets removed to the edges of the city, and the numbers of taverns, alehouses and tobacco shops reduced. The quality of the air was important, and could be improved if overcrowding was lessened and bad buildings in alleys, housing poor people, were demolished. When plague appeared, householders could open their windows during the day, but must close them before sunset, and crowding was potentially harmful. Stray dogs and cats in the streets should be killed and, in a potentially important observation, he com-mented that rats, mice, weasels and other vermin running from house to house could carry the infection and must be destroyed, while the citizens ought not to be permitted to keep tame rabbits and pigeons.

The advice which Mayerne provided was a comprehensive summary of current opinion; much of what he and the College recommended was familiar to the Council and many of the measures already were in force. Shortly before it was received, in March, the Council strengthened its policy by ordering the

Lord Mayor and justices that, although in London infected houses were closed for a month, in future the period should be forty days, 'as is used in other countryes and found by experience to be the safer coursse'. But some of the other proposals were not implemented. Even though some members of the committee which considered them would have approved of Mayerne's assertion that 'Order is the soule & life of all thinges', such order was difficult to achieve in Carolean London. The board of health and divisions into health districts would cut across existing jurisdictions and require an adequate and reliable source of funding. In the past, the corporation and county justices had shown a distinct reluctance to provide money unless it could be directly targeted at the victims of the disease, and the notion of financing a permanent and independent health establishment would not have been welcome. The king's hospital was not built, nor were the pesthouses. The urgency and concern which an outbreak of plague engendered faded again, for only 274 victims died of the disease in London during 1631 and the death toll over the next four years was just nine.

The College of Physicians did not take a lead and became distracted by a dispute with the apothecaries, who had broken away from the Grocers' Company in 1617. They had then been constituted as a separate company, and had continued to supply prescriptions during the plague in 1625, while the physicians had attracted obloquy because so many of them had left. Their absence during the epidemic had helped to weaken the College's direction of medical services in the capital, but during the early 1630s it attempted to reassert its control over the apothecaries, by requiring the members of their company to take a stricter oath. And the apothecaries were told by Mayerne to dispense the prescriptions set down by the physicians and not abuse the powers which they had been granted, but to 'use them with order, modesty, and reverence to their superiors, the physicians'. The College also claimed that the apothecaries' wares had to be submitted to it to be tested and approved – in other words, that they could not be trusted to supply medicines without supervision – and the physicians attempted to enforce this requirement.

Their actions related not only to precedent and the College maintaining its supremacy, but also showed a real concern that, without proper control, counterfeit medicines would be sold by those unqualified to prepare them. Such people were not above selling the 'most filthy concoctions, and even mud, under the name and title of medicaments'. The College's *Pharmacopia Londinensis* was a dispensatory which set out those prescriptions which were permitted, specified how apothecaries were to prepare medicines and contained those appropriate for treating and preventing plague. They included *theriac Londinensis*, or London Treacle, the recipe for which was attributed to an apothecary named Walsh, who had a shop in Holborn. This consisted of a blend of herbs soaked in a solution of three parts Malaga wine and one part honey, with a dram of opium, and was very popular – perhaps not surprisingly, given its ingredients.

Disputes within the medical professions were matched by disagreements over the administration of London. Because of its divided government, the Privy Council had to act as co-ordinator of the actions of the corporation and the county justices, and it attempted to resolve the problem with the incorporation of the suburbs in 1636. This was resented rather than welcomed by the City, which disliked the creation of a separate and potentially rival authority. Even so, in 1637 the Council still hoped that the aldermen would supervise the area covered by the new Corporation of the Suburbs in a commission of the peace, because of 'the great need for magistrates in those places in the time of plague'. But these arrangements proved to be a source of contention between the City and Charles I's government.

The City also disliked the policy of permitting houses built in defiance of the ban on new building to remain, on payment of a fine, effectively allowing bad environmental conditions to develop in order to raise revenue. In 1639, the Lord Mayor produced a list which showed that 1,361 such houses had been erected since 1603, only fifty-seven of them within his jurisdiction, but with 618 to the west of the City, 404 to the north and 282 to the east. Such expansion increased overcrowding and the problem of governing those areas, which worsened further when the unpopular Star Chamber Court was abolished by Parliament in 1641. According to the inhabitants of Westminster and the suburbs, this made matters more difficult by effectively producing an absence of government in their areas.

Some aspects of plague policy were accepted, such as the connection between disease and the fetid air produced by environmental pollution. This had been used to justify the orders against new building and overcrowding in London that had been issued since the first proclamation in 1580. The risks posed by a dirty and hence odiferous environment extended to the poor people who lived in such surroundings. A petition to the Council in 1632 complained of newly built tenements around the City, both north and south of the river, which brought beggars, pollution, higher prices for food and the danger of plague. An area of Clerkenwell surveyed in 1635 displayed the characteristics regarded as typical of such a district, both in the condition of the buildings and the habits of those who lived in them. Some of the houses were close to collapse and most of them were 'pore Raskoly habitations and Inhabited with Such like people for the most part'. They threw their rubbish, including dead cats and dogs, into the alleys, 'which in a contagious or infectious Tyme of Sicknes is very dangerous' for those living nearby. The conclusion was that 'unlesse that kind of people be Rowted from that place it wilbe both dangerous and unholsom to com neare them at Any tyme'. The logical, albeit brutal, solution which was recommended was the eviction of the occupants and demolition of the buildings. Here, at least, social prejudice dovetailed with plague policy.

Such attempts to clean up the polluted suburbs did not lead to a relaxation of vigilance regarding the threat from abroad. In 1635, the Privy Council became alarmed at the epidemics in Amsterdam, Leiden and Dunkirk. In 1635 and 1636, there were more than 25,000 deaths in Amsterdam and almost a third of the population of Leiden died. Anzolo Correr, the Venetian ambassador in London, reported to the Doge and Senate in October that the Council was concerned about the outbreaks on the continent, yet it would not take any action for fear of harming trade. The Council had warned the merchants to be cautious, but, as he pointed out, it was not the habit of merchants to do anything to damage their own commercial interests.

In fact, the Council had asked the corporation for advice, which was rather strange, as the quarantining of shipping was an integral part of its own policy, implemented a few years earlier, and it, not the Lord Mayor and aldermen, had the authority to impose the restriction. Nevertheless, they did respond, with the recommendation that vessels should require a licence from the customs officers before they could land passengers or cargo, that officers should board incoming vessels to prevent anyone or anything being taken off, and that ships from infected places should not be granted permission to discharge people or goods for 'some certain days'. The Council acted on this, and a proclamation was issued accordingly 'to restraine the landing of Goods, or comming ashore of Men out of such Shipping, untill due tryall shall bee had, that the same may bee done without perill or danger of Infection'. Correr approved of the policy, but commented that it should have been introduced sooner.

Strict implementation of the quarantine proved to be difficult. In one incident, a French nobleman and his suite arrived at Great Yarmouth from Brielle, in Holland, and were allowed to land on condition that they occupied a house that was allocated to them, until they had served the period of quarantine. They ignored the restriction, obtained some horses, rode to London and even appeared at court, before the Council was aware that the quarantine had been breached. In April 1636, while the number of plague deaths in the Bills was still small, the officers at Gravesend reported that they had detained a ship from Rotterdam, but that the watermen were not being co-operative. More concerned with making money than observing the regulations, they had boarded the ship and had been hired by the passengers, probably to take them to London. The officers had been powerless to prevent this and, indeed, could only enforce the regulations with much danger and trouble to themselves.

In any case, from whatever source, the disease had reached London, and the number of deaths reported in the Bills was beginning to increase, especially in the eastern suburbs. The returns were the most comprehensive yet, with the addition of seven parishes, on both sides of the river, in the middle of April. This did not please the corporation, which petitioned the king:

> …that his majesty will be pleased, that all those which die of the plague in the parish of Stepney may not be certified in the weekly bills of London, as his majesty hath commanded lately, but that they may be certified in a bill by itself; because, it being included in the city bills, it is generally taken abroad that London is more infected than, God be thanked, it is: so it not only breeds a fear in the country-people of coming to London, but of receiving any commodities from the city.

Such fear of an epidemic grew, especially with the warm weather at the end of April, and Correr predicted a large-scale evacuation of the city if the numbers continued to rise. The plague orders were reissued, and on 22 April an order was made for the building of pesthouses and 'other places of abode' for the victims, continuing the policy promoted by the Council in 1625 of housing the sick in hut encampments. Before the end of the month, the justices of the Tower Division reported that they had closed all houses where plague victims lived, had set guards to watch them night and day, and appointed searchers, sextons and bearers. Provisions were supplied to those incarcerated, with a tax of £100 imposed on every parish for the purpose; they had allocated sites for building huts and sheds to which the sick could be taken, and had also pursued the longer-term objective of prosecuting householders who were contributing to overcrowding by taking in lodgers.

Towards the end of May, those incarcerated in the debtors' prisons became alarmed, as the disease began to spread, and they petitioned the king for their release, which he granted, as he had done in 1625. On 13 May, Sir John Burgh wrote that the number of plague deaths had risen in the previous week to fifty-five, which 'breeds a great terror'. A week later, Viscount Chaworth took a more rational line, admitting that 'apprehension of the Plague' was greater than ever, although in his opinion the disease was 'not considerable'. His lodgings were in the Strand, which naturally influenced his perception of the danger, for on 10 June he could write that the Bill 'was this month 87 in all Stepney & those parishes'. The citizens were more afraid than 'the better sort' and he estimated that at least 4,000 people had already left London. Unusually, during the spring the plague claimed victims in more than one of the houses belonging to members of the aristocracy, which may have shaken the complacency of those in and around Whitehall. Careful observers would have noted that the increase in plague deaths was uneven, with three weeks in May, June and July showing a significant fall in the numbers recorded, but doubts arose about the accuracy of the recording, expressed in plain terms as 'more die than are certified'. Archbishop William Laud's secretary, William Dell, thought that in the large parish of St Botolph-without-Bishopsgate there had been twenty-two deaths in one week, twelve of them plague victims, yet only four had been entered in that category.

In the case reported by Dell, the total number of deaths was accurately returned, but the figure for plague deaths had been falsified. Not until the last week of July did the returns for all deaths begin to increase significantly; the 1,375 burials recorded in the four weeks of July were outstripped by the 2,454 entered in August, and the number continued to rise. The week ending 15 September had 1,306 deaths and the following one 1,229, but hopes that this marked the beginning of a decline were to be disappointed, for the last week of September saw 1,403 deaths and the first week of October two more than that. Five Bills were issued during September, with a total of 6,018 deaths, and four in October, which showed 4,609 deaths. The numbers attributed to plague followed the same pattern as the total, peaking in the last week of September and the first week of October, when sixty-six per cent were entered in that category. The expected decline during the autumn was slow, with deaths from all causes in the last week of November being higher than in even the highest week in August, and not until early December did the number of recorded plague victims fall below half of the total deaths.

Despite the slow progress of the epidemic in the early summer, by the middle of June the exodus of citizens to towns around the capital had produced overcrowding problems, with two or three families living in one house, which was identified as a potential risk if the plague should spread to them. These were short-term lodgers, who would leave when the epidemic declined, and displacing them could only move the problem elsewhere. But enforced removal of potential carriers of plague had become a feature of the Council's policy. Four days after his accession, the king had ordered that rogues, vagabonds, beggars and prostitutes loitering at the gates of Whitehall Palace should be removed, reflecting his fastidious nature, which contrasted with that of his father, as well as concern about the danger of contagion which dirty people were thought to represent. The displacement of those regarded as posing a health risk was adopted by the Council as a means of protecting the royal household when plague threatened in 1636.

Some Londoners sent their children to schools at Enfield, Waltham and other places close to the royal palace at Theobalds, and they or their servants visited them there, which was seen as a potential danger, and the Council required that they should be removed. The numbers of houses held by Londoners in and around Kingston, Teddington and Isleworth were considered to increase the risk of plague reaching the palaces of Hampton Court, Nonsuch and Oatlands. The Council responded by prohibiting anyone from travelling to them from the capital, at the risk of being removed from the houses or quarantined within them. In September, it noted that refugees from the capital had brought the plague to Eltham, near the palace there, and it also ordered the evacuation of Londoners from houses within six miles of Windsor Castle. The size of the areas specified and the potential numbers of people involved must have made it difficult to implement these orders, which may reflect Charles I's anxiety rather than an attempt to impose an effective plague policy. But the solution to the problem of protecting the royal family from plague now involved the quarantining or removal of people from considerable areas around a number of royal palaces, and was far removed from Henry VIII's response of skulking almost alone in the country-side for his own safety.

More easily enforceable were the bans on the fairs in and around London. The wisdom of the policy was questioned, for it did not deter the country people from bringing their produce and livestock to be sold, or trading in the villages around the city, rather than at the fairs, where it could be regulated more easily. The bans were enforced, nevertheless, for prohibiting people from assembling in large groups remained one of the measures taken to prevent the spread of plague, although church services were again treated as exceptions. In October, a general weekly fast was ordered and a form of service was issued to the clergy, with the instruction that they should detain the congregation no longer than the time it took to conduct the service, 'because such detaining of the people so long together, may prove dangerous to the further increase of the Sicknesse'. Public performances of plays, entertainments and sports were prohibited altogether, but this was not fully observed, for a bear-baiting which drew a large crowd said to number many thousands was held on 18 October at the Paris Garden at Bankside, the principal bear-baiting house in the capital, despite the ban.

Such defiant behaviour was familiar from previous epidemics, as were the problems that ensued from the quarantining of the sick and their contacts. These were due to the sheer numbers involved, and the cost. Maintaining just two quarantined families in St Sepulchre-without-Newgate cost the parish £10 17s 3d. In St Martin's-in-the-Fields, the 324 houses which were closed contained 388 families consisting of 1,328 people; the parish of St Botolph-without-Bishopsgate, which held approximately 6,000 communicants, received only a small sum from the Lord Mayor; and thousands of people in Southwark were reported to be in 'great necessity'. The Privy Council had to remind the Surrey justices that to aid the victims in Southwark they were entitled to levy a tax on the whole county, as provided for in the Plague Act of 1604. Yet they must have been aware that in the circumstances assessing a tax was far easier than collecting the money, especially in the parishes fringing London. In Holborn £40 had been assessed, but no more than £2 was likely to be received before the epidemic came to an end. Inadequate funds may have contributed to the familiar problem, reported to the Lord Mayor, of 'beggars, rogues, wanderers, and dissolute persons', some with plague sores, openly roaming around the streets, despite the quarantine measures.

One way in which the poor could raise some money was by selling clothes to the dealers in rags, who supplied the paper-makers. The rag dealers bought clothes cheaply from the poor and then stored them in cellars on their premises in the suburbs around the northern fringes of the city. Textiles were thought to be one of the ways in which plague was disseminated, and so the trade attracted the attention of the justices. While they had the authority to arrest and punish the dealers as 'rogues', they needed authority to seize and destroy the stocks of rags. This could be done most easily and quickly by burning them, but with the risk of spreading the plague by infecting the air. Burying the rags was safer, yet, perhaps surprisingly, the Privy Council preferred that they should be burnt. It attempted to stop the trade in rags and old clothes by cutting demand, when it ordered that the paper mills should stop operating during the epidemic. The ramifications of an outbreak of plague were far-reaching.

In October, a John Eliot wrote from his house near the Savoy to Sir John Coke, one of the Secretaries of State, complaining that the plague orders were being disobeyed and noting that many people continued to go to funerals. He feared the lawlessness that had arisen from the departure of all those in authority, with 'many thousands' of dubious characters in the suburbs who lived 'by the spoil' of others. Apprentices and servants were in want because their masters had left, and the absence of the justices had contributed to the increase in the numbers of beggars, rogues and vagabonds. Among those who had suffered from the downturn in business during the epidemic were the watermen, porters, coachmen, tailors, shoemakers, glovers, silk-weavers and 'discarded Irish footmen'. He recommended the appointment of a City Marshal to tackle the problems, with power to go through the suburbs to root out the vagrants, and was brave enough to enclose a draft warrant for his own appointment to the post. Problems produced by plague brought opportunities as well as disruption.

Another potential danger to which he drew attention was the threat of violence directed against the French community. Papers had been strewn about the streets warning of the destruction of all French people in London. Such hostility to immigrants was not especially unusual and normally would not have carried much risk of disorder, but foreign communities operated independently of the parochial arrangements and the resentment which they attracted was more likely to erupt into violence during epidemics. In the middle of April, the writer of a letter from London reported that:

> The last week, there died of the plague, two French children out of one house, in Whitechapel parish. Upon search, since, it appears that in Stepney and Whitechapel, eight houses have been infected, and fifteen persons have died of the plague, and all French, as I hear.

This suggested deliberate concealment of the disease, which was likely to arouse hostility, as it delayed the implementation of quarantine and other countermeasures. Antipathy was expressed by those in authority as well as the citizenry. The justices of the Tower Division had reported that when they distributed assistance to those in quarantined households, they had not given any to the members of the French congregation.

To overcome their exclusion from the system of relief, the French-Walloon and Dutch congregations, which contained roughly 1,400 and 840 members respectively, appointed 'consolators' to take alms and comfort to the sick or bereaved. To fulfil their duties, they had to visit houses where plague victims lived and then go around the streets and mix with others. In doing so, they disobeyed the quarantine orders for the closing of houses and incarceration of those who visited the infected. The Dutch consistory at Austin Friars appointed a visitor of the sick, but as early as May was aware of the problems which he would face and approached the French-Walloon community to discover if it had received relevant information from the corporation.

For their part, in June the Privy Councillors instructed the justices to warn the 'consolators' that infected houses should be closed and that if they continued with their existing pattern, they would be confined in them. Despite the members' earlier anxiety about the regulations, the consistory was now defiant and agreed that the visitor should continue to act 'in accordance with God', a higher authority than the corporation or the Council. The crisis placed a severe strain on the consistory's relief funds, especially as 'the wealthier members have taken up their residences in the countryside'. When an extra collection was required, they were contacted and asked for contributions, even if they were not willing to return in person. The collection raised £803, which did something to restore the poor relief funds. The outlay in 1636 was £2,860, compared with £1,530 in 1635.

Among those who were recommended to the deacons for help was the schoolmaster, whose fee-paying pupils had ceased to attend because of the risk of infection, leaving him impoverished. Eventually, the corporation ordered the closure of all of the schools in the City. The school of Thomas Sutton's charity at the Charterhouse was also at risk because 'many

Towne Boyes and Outcommers from divers parts of the Citty and Suburbs are received and taught in the hospitall Schoole' and so it, too, was closed. This had been provided for in the charity's statutes, promulgated in 1627, which directed that during an epidemic scholars with parents or friends nearby should be sent to them, and those 'destitute of friends or means, they shall be sent out and maintained by the hospital'. Similar provision was made for the almsmen, but those too infirm or elderly to leave were to remain in the almshouse, where they were to be cared for by 'two elder grooms to make the provisions, and three old women lodged in the house'. The rules were evidently compiled in the belief that the elderly were less likely to succumb to plague.

London's Roman Catholics faced a similar challenge, in providing relief for those who were excluded from help from the parishes, yet keeping within the plague regulations. Cecily Crowe, of Bloomsbury, later objected that the parish would not make donations to recusants, despite the fact that Catholic families contributed to the parish rate for the plague victims. But the poor Catholics did not observe the other orders, especially the rule that infected houses should be sealed, for they believed it to be 'a matter of conscience to visit their neighbours in any sickness, yea, though they know it to be infection; even the red cross does not keep them out'.

Matthew Wilson, Superior of the London Jesuits, and the chapter of the secular clergy each appointed a representative to care for the plague victims. The clergy chose Fr John Southworth, and Wilson's choice was Fr Henry Morse, who since 1633 had been based in St Giles-in-the-Fields. Wearing a 'distinctive mark' on his clothing and carrying a white rod, throughout the epidemic Morse busied himself in visiting the sick in rooms that were 'oppressive with foul and pestilential air', acquiring medicines for them, providing bedding and clothes to replace those which had been burnt, hearing confessions and laying out the dead. When those guarding the closed houses refused to allow the priests to enter, the money was handed over at the windows. Morse visited Protestant as well as Catholic families, and some of those he had helped later testified to his dedication. Elizabeth Godwin of St Giles, who described herself as 'a poor labouring woman', was incarcerated in her house for seven weeks and three of her children died, and Morse helped her 'with her Majesty's and with divers Catholics' alms'. Despite the queen's contributions to the relief fund, the expense was so great that in October, when they were still trying to support around fifty families, the two priests had to appeal beyond London to Catholics across England, because of 'the extreame necessity which many of the poorer sort are fallen into'.

Their appeal stressed just how bad the disaster was; indeed, it was so awful that they would not have believed it if they had not seen it for themselves and experienced its effects every day. To encourage donations, they pointed out how well the Protestants had responded to the crisis: one nobleman had donated £300 and the son of one of the aldermen had visited those in need and made donations. And they painted a gloomy picture of the conditions which those who were quarantined had to endure:

> There are some persons in the number of these afflicted, who, notwithstanding they were well borne, and bred, having beene constrained, through extremity of want, to sell, or pawne all they had, remaine shut up within the bare walls of a poore chamber, having not wherewithall to allay the rage of hunger, nor scarcely to cover nakednesse. There are others, who, for the space of three dayes togeather have not gotten a morsell of bread to put into their mouths. Wee have just cause to feare, that some doe perish for want of food: others for want of [at]tendance: others for want of ordinary helpes and remedies.

Neither of the priests succumbed to plague, but both were arrested, Southworth at the end of October and Morse in February 1637. After four weeks in Newgate, Morse was brought to trial and found guilty, but on the intervention of the king he was released in June.

By the time of Morse's arrest, the epidemic had declined. The Bills recorded 23,359 deaths during 1636, 10,400 of which were attributed to plague. The increased mortality in the City parishes was relatively small, but St Giles Cripplegate, St Botolph-without-Bishopsgate and St Botolph-without-Aldgate experienced an almost fourfold rise in deaths. These were the areas where members of the foreign communities were concentrated, and their burials were not recorded in the parish registers, so the true numbers of deaths in those parishes may have been higher than the figures indicate. St Martin's-in-the-Fields also suffered severely, with an increase from thirteen burials in March to seventy-two in July, seventy-five in August and 101 in September, when the registers break off. The epidemic, although not as severe as those in 1603 or 1625, showed a similar pattern to them, with a relatively low incidence of plague deaths in the centre and a high impact on the suburbs, especially those on the north and north-east sides of the City.

The epidemic continued into 1637, and prompted an order of the Privy Council designed to limit the effects of the outbreak of the previous year. This was read in the churches on a Sunday early in January and ordered:

> That all such householders as had lived in the country all the time of the infection, whose houses in and about the city had been infected, these were forbidden to return to their houses before the next justice of the peace should give way to it; which he shall not do until he be assured that those same infected houses, and all the stuff in them, have been

thoroughly aired; for, indeed, the want of this care hath been
the cause of the increase of the plague in some of these last
weeks. Also, no lodgers are to be admitted this next term in
any of these said infected houses, but by the next justice of
peace's approbation.

Despite such measures, during 1637, 3,082 plague deaths were
recorded among a total of 11,723 burials from all causes, the
highest figure for the disease since 1625, with the sole exception of 1636. Baptisms showed a slight decline in 1637, when
they were four per cent fewer than in 1636 and nine per cent
fewer than in 1635. The metropolis now had a population that
exceeded 300,000, and the number of burials averaged 11,730
during the late 1630s, including 363 plague deaths in 1638 and
314 in 1639. Other English cities suffered epidemics during
these years, including Newcastle-upon-Tyne, Hull, Norwich
and Leicester. An outbreak in 1637 at Worcester was the worst
since the mid-sixteenth century, killing about ten per cent of
the city's population.

Plague in London and elsewhere brought a decline in trade,
as English goods were quarantined or banned in other countries. Spain prohibited all ships from London from entering
her ports, and those from Dover, which had developed as the
centre of a lucrative entrepôt trade, were subject to a quarantine period of forty days. An agreement with Spain concluded
in 1632 had produced a steady increase in the amount of silver
coined at the Mint, so that from a modest 1,629lbs in 1631 it
coined 88,089lbs in 1635, but this was checked in 1636, which
saw a fall to 42,418lbs. Because of the interruption caused by
the plague, the Spanish authorities diverted the supplies for the
Army of Flanders through Italy and along the Spanish Road to
the Low Countries. The effect was so serious that early in 1637
Lord Aston, the English ambassador in Spain, tried to persuade
them to permit the reopening of trade with London, but he

was not successful. The deaths from plague of three people in the household of the Spanish ambassador in London, in March 1637, did little to encourage the lifting of the ban. Eventually, with French armies blocking the overland route to Flanders from Italy, and the falling number of deaths from the disease recorded in the London Bills, the Spanish relented, and on 1 November Aston reported that their ports would be reopened. The trade in goods and silver recommenced and recovered; in 1638, the silver coined at the Mint was almost double the weight processed in 1635, at 169,387lbs, but the epidemic had disrupted an important sector of the English economy for over a year.

Despite such disruption, during the 1630s both London and the economy escaped the kind of problems brought to much of the continent by plague and war, until those dangers began to loom larger, with the two Bishops' Wars between England and Scotland in 1639 and 1640, the rebellion in Ireland, which began in 1641, and the outbreak of the English Civil War in 1642. These resulted in the greater movement of people – soldiers, camp followers, suppliers and refugees – and the weakening of civilian administration, as the military increasingly took wider powers. London was the Parliamentarian headquarters and principal supply base; its citizens served as soldiers and the City's militia campaigned with the Parliamentarian armies.

The Civil War also caused an influx of people to London from around the British Isles – not, as in peacetime, predominantly the young people who provided many of the immigrants to the metropolis and took up apprenticeships or places as servants, but those displaced by the war, who arrived penniless. By the summer of 1645, there were twelve refugee families in a house in Whitecross Street that belonged to Sir Robert Foster, a Justice of the Common Pleas and a Royalist. But they were not squatters; they had been assigned space there. Foster had moved to Oxford, Charles I's headquarters, and his house had been requisitioned to provide homes for refugees. These included people from Bristol, 'driven from their habitation', a family 'driven by the king's forces from Salisbury', two brothers 'plundered and driven away from Staffordshire', a man from Wells in Somerset 'driven away by the enemy', others from Berkshire, Lyme Regis, Tetbury in Gloucestershire, and a widow from County Cavan, who was told that she could live in the kitchen, with use of a closet. Jane Beck and her three children were allocated a 'low room in the inner garden' and a little cellar. The war had been unkind to Jane. Her husband had joined the Parliamentarian cavalry, but had been killed at York. As if that was not bad enough, the house in Birmingham where she and her children lived was one of eighty or more burnt down by the Royalists when they captured the town in May 1643. After these misfortunes, she had brought the children to London for safety and was facing eviction when she was placed in Foster's house.

It surely would have been unthinkable just a few years earlier that the house of a senior lawyer would be packed full of destitute people. Yet this experience was repeated across London, with the empty mansions of other absent Royalists providing rooms for those displaced by the fighting. Mary Searle had come from Exeter, where she looked after sick and wounded Parliamentarian soldiers, and Dorothy Salway had travelled from Worcestershire, where she had been plundered, losing all her goods.

The refugees also included those clergymen and members of their congregations who took evasive action because their puritan convictions were unpalatable to the Royalists. William Taylor was rector of Cirencester, but moved to London after that town was sacked by the king's troops in 1643. John Tombes, the vicar of Leominster, first went to Bristol and then, following its capture by the Royalists in July 1643, moved to London. Walter Cradock and members of his church at Llanvaches in

Monmouthshire did the same. Another clergyman, Nicholas Staughton, had come only from Surrey, fleeing to London when Royalist forces burst into the county in November 1642.

With the outbreak of war, controls on admittance were put in place, and in the spring of 1643 the city was surrounded by a line of earthwork fortifications, which allowed access to be controlled as never before, with checkpoints at the gates in the line. This should have made it possible to exclude those who were from areas infected by plague and did not have health certificates, but normal economic life had to continue and Parliament's own troops and supporters could not be refused admission. The refugees who arrived had to be housed in the already overcrowded city, producing conditions which the authorities regarded as conducive to plague, with subdivided properties and a polluted environment generating foul air. Some were treated in the hospitals. Within three years, Bridewell Hospital admitted almost 2,900 'wandering soldiers, cavalier-prisoners, and other vagrants'.

The number of plague burials had increased before the outbreak of the Civil War, with 1,450 deaths attributed to the disease in 1640 and a rise in the numbers during the following summer, which alarmed the members of the Long Parliament. This was not a rapidly developing epidemic. Deaths were recorded in Chancery Lane and Holborn by the middle of July and in Westminster a month later. Nevertheless, it gave rise to some concern, with Sir Simonds D'Ewes deciding that he should find new lodgings, in cleaner air, and the Commons agreeing without question to grant leave of absence to Members who were thought to have had contact with plague victims.

An order of the Commons on 26 August directed that the houses where infected people had been quarantined should be marked, guarded and 'safely locked up'. The justices for

Middlesex and Westminster wondered about the extent of their own authority while Parliament was sitting, and eleven days later asked for a conference with the Commons to decide how to deal with the plague cases. Until this was held, they delayed implementing the plague orders, which clearly had a lower priority with the justices than ensuring that the correct protocol was observed. On 8 September, the orders were agreed by both Houses, the day before Parliament was adjourned. Evidently, speed of execution had not been the main concern.

Plague made a much more dramatic impact when, after the sitting was resumed, it was the weapon employed in an assassination attempt on the life of the Parliamentarian leader John Pym. On 25 October, a porter was given a package to take to him in the House of Commons, with the instruction that it should be opened in the Chamber. When Pym unsealed it, a dirty and bloody rag fell out, identified as a plaster from a plague sore, along with a letter warning him that if the contagion did not kill him, a dagger would be used. A suspect was arrested shortly afterwards, but when he was questioned was found not to be responsible and so was released. Pym and the other Members in the Commons at the time survived unharmed, having been given both a fright and an opportunity that could be exploited for propaganda purposes. The writer of the pamphlet which broke the news of this 'Divellish, and Unchristian Plot against the High Court of Parliament' did not hesitate to blame Roman Catholics, who were believed to employ assassination as an instrument of policy, asking rhetorically 'what rationall man in the world will not say, that such Popish Inventions come from the Divell?'.

The epidemic had continued its steady course throughout September, with the number of deaths reaching around 300 a week, and peaked in the first week of October. A few days after the plague plaster was delivered to the Commons, the House ordered that the justices for London, Westminster and Middlesex should ensure that the Ordinance issued two months earlier was being strictly enforced. By then the disease was receding, but it caused a recorded 3,210 plague deaths during the year, including those in the 'distant parishes', which was the highest since 1637.

The outbreak had been serious enough to prompt suggestions that Parliament should adjourn to the relative safety of Oxford. This would have had a major political impact, moving it away from the London crowds which supported Pym and provided a refuge for the Crown's opponents, which was to be dramatically demonstrated in the following January, when Charles attempted to arrest the five Members who he thought were orchestrating the opposition to him. The suggested move to Oxford was one of the reasons which prompted Louis du Moulin to prepare a paper for the House of Commons. The son of a French Protestant minister, du Moulin had been educated at Leiden, had come to England in 1630 and was licenced by the College of Physicians in 1640.

Du Moulin's main point was that adequate plague prevention measures would contain outbreaks, forestalling the 'huge and fearfull increase' in the number of deaths, removing the need for Parliament to sit elsewhere and avoiding 'the great decay of trading' in London. He favoured the implementation of the proposals by the College of Physicians and Mayerne for a permanent health board. Now that the period of the king's personal rule had come to an end, the Commons could take the initiative and order that they should be put in place, with doctors, surgeons and apothecaries, appointed and approved by the College, allocated for treating plague victims. They would be sworn to visit anyone, attending the poor 'for God's sake' and the 'abler sort' for the usual fees. This should be done before an epidemic began; once one had erupted, it was too late to implement such arrangements. Having dedicated plague doctors freed the other members of the medical profession from attending its victims, and reduced the risk of them spreading the disease by visiting both plague sufferers and those who were free from it. To compensate the members of the plague board for the loss of their usual practice, and for the risks which they ran, he suggested generous rates of remuneration and pensions for their widows equivalent to a third of their salaries. He recognised, too, the need for spiritual comfort for victims, as well as medical treatment, and commented that it was 'to be expected and wished That the Bishopp of the dioces should during the Infection appoint Ministers to visitt the Infected'.

The scheme required funding of at least £1,100 annually for salaries alone, which could be raised by contributions from the City and surrounding districts that produced £2,500 per annum, the equivalent of 3d per house, based on an estimate of 50,000 houses. This would overcome the difficulty of trying to collect rates during an epidemic, which had again been obvious during the epidemic in 1636. Unspent sums could be used to build new pesthouses and enlarge the existing ones.

These proposals were a cogent summary of current thinking, similar to those put forward by the College and Mayerne, and suggested solutions to the practical problems, but they were not implemented. The physicians' relations with the other two branches of the medical profession were still unsettled, and du Moulin's financial arrangements, although neat, probably were impracticable. The City had always been opposed to such perpetual levies for plague care. In 1636, the Privy Council had expressed the fear that the numbers of poor had increased so much that the wealthy were unable to provide relief for them during normal years, 'much less' during an epidemic, with the consequence that those who were unwell had to mix with the healthy. A constant tax of the kind proposed would be a burden on those citizens who were well enough off to have to pay it.

Parliament was no more willing or able to impose such an arrangement than the Privy Council had been ten years earlier. Both Houses were preoccupied with more pressing political and military matters and, in any case, the threat of a plague epidemic was much less in 1642 than in the previous year, with 1,373 plague deaths, fewer than half the number for 1641. And, although plague was present throughout the years of the first Civil War, at no time did an epidemic threaten to develop on the scale of that in 1636, with the number of deaths from plague between 1642 and 1646 averaging fewer than 2,000 per year. Even so, plague continued to be a cause of anxiety for Londoners. No doubt mindful of his daughter's death in the epidemic of 1625, when Nehemiah Wallington suddenly fell sick he at once thought that he had 'bine strock with the plauge', although that proved not to be the case. John Greene, a lawyer lodging in Old Jewry, kept an anxious eye on the Bills during those years, especially in May 1644, when plague was identified in three or four houses in his own parish, with two or three deaths in each of the infected houses. And in the West End, Thomas Gunning lost his wife and three children to plague, and he only recovered after an illness that lasted for sixteen weeks.

The number of plague deaths increased again in 1646, as the war came to an end, despite a severe winter during which the Thames above London Bridge froze over. In August, the plague orders were reissued, with the observation that 'there hath beene heretofore great abuse in misreporting the disease'. To help overcome this, someone who was taken ill was to be suspected of suffering from plague unless the symptoms were clearly those of another disease. And the speed of response was important; when anyone developed a 'Botch, or Purple, or Swelling in any part of his body, or falleth otherwise danger-ously sick, without apparent cause of some other disease' then the head of the household was to report the case to one of the examiners within two hours of the symptoms appearing. Officers were to be appointed, the quarantined houses marked and a weekly rate collected. Among the causes blamed for the spread of the disease were the sale of putrid fish, musty corn and rotten flesh and fruit, as well as those familiar targets, the 'disorderly Tipling in Tavernes Ale houses and Cellers... the common sinne of this time and greatest occasion of dispersing the Plague', and the many rogues and wandering beggars 'that swarm in every place about the City'. Playhouses were not mentioned; they had been closed in 1642 and were not to reopen until after the restoration of the monarchy in 1660.

The epidemic in 1646 was not severe enough to cause the cancellation of Bartholomew Fair, despite the 2,567 plague burials recorded during the year, almost seventeen per cent of the total. The disease was more virulent in 1647, when the figure for plague burials was much higher, at 3,951, which represented twenty-four per cent of all interments. But it declined thereafter, with 693 plague burials in 1648, and just seventy-one in 1649, and throughout the 1650s the number of deaths from the disease was negligible. In four years, they were in single figures, and the highest number for a year during the decade was thirty-six, in 1659. John Milton deployed this as an argument against restoring the monarchy. In *The Ready and Easy Way to establish a Free Commonwealth* (1660), he countered the popular view that only the return of the Stuarts could revive trade, with the comment that people had forgotten 'the frequent Plagues and Pestilences that then wasted this City, such as through God's Mercy we never have felt' since the establishment of the republic. With the low numbers of plague deaths, facilities intended for its victims could be put to other uses. After the battle of Worcester in 1651, the inhabitants of Westminster were paid £30 by the Council of State 'for repairing the pest house and churchyard where the Scotch prisoners were kept'.

The figures from the Bills were collected and analysed by John Graunt in a pioneering study of London's demography, published in 1662 as *Natural and Political Observations... upon the Bills of Mortality*. He examined a range of characteristics of the metropolis's population, including the reasons for its growth, commenting on the insufficient number of births to maintain its size and hence its reliance on immigration from the country, the causes of death and the periodic bursts of high mortality. He regarded a plague year as one in which the number of deaths from the disease exceeded 200, and his calculations to assess which of the epidemic years had been the worst, allowing for the growing population, suggested that the outbreaks in 1603 and 1625 had been equally destructive, with one fifth of the population dying in each outbreak. He estimated that under-registration of deaths from plague was of the order of twenty-five per cent in 1625 and 1636, by comparing the number of deaths in those years with the average for the immediately preceding and succeeding years.

Graunt did not accept that plague was contagious and believed that it 'depends more upon the Disposition of the Air, than upon the Effluvia from the Bodies of men'. This explained the rapid variation in numbers of deaths, which must be due to changes in the air, not the constitution of people's bodies, and so household quarantine was 'not a remedy to be purchased at vast inconveniences'. He concluded that all outbreaks of 'acute and Epidemical Diseases' were caused by such 'corruptions and alterations in the Air'.

Yet the author of a submission to the government written at about the same time, suggesting 'some few Expedients for the Prevention of the Plague', was sure that the disease 'for the most part is spread by Contact & Infection... hinder the Contact & you prevent the Infection'. Previous practices had been at fault and had even contributed to the extent of the disease:

That which hath rendred all meanes hitherto provided against the Plague inefectuall, is, the particular reguard to the Cure, & the totall Neglect of the Prevention, which is the Principall & belongs to the Magistrate; and indeed the late usuall Methods & Practises have been so farr from lessening or preventing the Plague, that it hath very much augmented & promoted it, the fear of its Consequent mischiefs, necessitating the Infected to Conceale their Infection . . . The Present Practice is, To shutt up no house 'till some is dead of the Plague, which oft-times by Bribery escapes unknown: but if knowne; too late, for possibly severall Visitants are by this time infected in divers Places, but when it shall be published That every infected Person shall have Physitian, Chirurgeon, Medicines, sufficient Attendance and Plentyfull Allowance dureing their sicknesse, and satisfaction for the losse of Time & Spoyle of Goods att the Common charge; 'tis not likely that many then will conceale their misfortune, and 'tis much better & cheaper for the Publick to make this provision for a few Houses, than to have that generall Confusion, that was in the last Plague, for want of it, for 40 houses well provided for, may prevent the Infection of 10000.

This latest proposal to make household quarantine more amenable to those who were to be confined would have been expensive, even if it did succeed in limiting the number of people affected. The author proposed that a fund be created in advance and 'some effectuall way for a speedy Collection of a sufficient summe' be devised, although this had not proved possible in the past. The expense included the 'good Salaries' for the members of the medical professions, who were 'to be at all times in a Readinesse'. They were to work with a group of commissioners, effectively forming a health board of the kind proposed in the 1630s, but, once again, the scheme was not implemented.

The danger of an epidemic was increasing because London was growing ever larger. Graunt estimated that its population was 460,000. Paris may have been slightly larger, but the other cities in northern Europe were much smaller. Amsterdam had grown rapidly since the late sixteenth century and probably had roughly 175,000 inhabitants by the 1650s, while Antwerp had 70,000 and Hamburg 75,000. Apart from Lisbon and Madrid, which each had 130,000 inhabitants, and Istanbul, the other European cities with populations in excess of 100,000 at that date were in Italy. Like many of his contemporaries, Graunt was concerned by London's growth, in both absolute and relative terms, and echoed a phrase of Sir Thomas Roe's, in 1641, when he described it as 'perhaps a Head too big for the Body'. He was also aware of the shift of focus westwards within the metropolis.

The development of the West End had not prevented over-crowding within the walls, where pressure on space had resulted in the conversion of the aristocracy's houses into tenements and the 'cramming up of the void spaces and Gardens within the Walls with Houses, to the prejudice of Light and Air'. Others commented on the consequences of London's growth, including Hugh Peter, the New Model Army's chaplain. He had spent some time in exile at Amsterdam before the Civil War and set his standards of cleanliness by the Dutch example. He complained of London's 'most beastly durtie streets', full of mud that fouled clothing and footwear and carried into houses. They should be paved with flat stones, with gutters along each side to drain them and raised footpaths of brick in front of the houses. The amount of horse-drawn traffic con-tributed to the problem, which could be reduced if measures were adopted to lessen the number of coaches coming into the city, and sleds should be used instead of carts, as in Amsterdam. The urban environment would also be improved if new houses were built of brick and stone, not timber, with wood used only for windows and doors. This would lessen the risk of fire and so encourage foreign merchants to store their goods in the city. In this respect, he anticipated the regulations issued to control the rebuilding after the Great Fire in 1666.

John Evelyn also criticised conditions in the capital. In *Fumifugium: Or The Inconveniencie of the Aer and Smoak of London Dissipated*, which was published in 1661, he complained of the 'Congestion of mishapen and extravagant Houses' and the spouts and gutters on the buildings, which were 'troublesome and malicious', so that when it had rained the water continued to cascade down, making it 'a continual Wet-day after the Storm is over'. He described the streets as 'narrow and incommodious in the very Center, and busiest places of Intercourse', with uneven paving, and, because of the rubbish which was daily thrown out of the houses, they were 'dirty even to a Proverb'. But Evelyn was more concerned with air pollution, which was caused by the 'poisonous and filthy Smoak' from domestic coal fires and, more especially, that from the premises of brewers, dyers, lime-burners, salt-makers and soap-boilers. Those of the butchers, tallow-chandlers and fishmongers also contributed to the problem and 'the frequency of Church-yards, and Charnel-Houses contamminate the Aer, in many parts of this town'.

Evelyn contrasted London's polluted atmosphere with the clean air in Paris, whose citizens predominantly used wood as a fuel, and suggested that this was a reason for its relative freedom from plague epidemics, while the venomous nature of coal smoke provided a means for the spread of 'Pestilential and Epidemical Sicknesses'. Graunt had a similar view, and thought that London was a less healthy place than it had been at the turn of the century because of the increasing use of coal. He believed that Newcastle was 'more unhealthful than other places' and that many people could not bear 'the smoak of London, not only for its unpleasantness, but for the suffocations which it causes'. The College of Physicians, on the other hand, regarded London's polluted air not as unhealthy but rather as 'a Preservation against Infections'. The fact that the incidence of plague was being discussed in such terms indicates that air quality was still thought to be a major factor in the spread of the disease. Yet, while there was general agreement that the bad air produced by putrefying rubbish, manure and stagnant water was dangerous, there was uncertainty as to whether the pollution produced by coal smoke protected a city against plague.

Despite such complaints about London's polluted environment, its citizens experienced few serious epidemics caused by diseases other than plagues. The rapid growth in its population was matched by an increase in supplies of food. Hardly anyone starved, a fact noted by Graunt, who pointed out that in his sample years of 1629–36 and 1647–58 only fifty-one of the 229,250 deaths in the Bills, just two-hundredths of one per cent, had been attributed to starvation. Water provision, too, had kept pace with population growth. In the early 1580s, the Dutchman Peter Morice had constructed a wheel that used the pressure of the flow through the arches at the north end of London Bridge to raise water as high as Leadenhall. In the mid-1590s, Bevis Bulmar constructed a similar arrangement at Broken Wharf, and in the 1650s a 'rare engine' designed by Sir Edward Ford could raise water from the river to a height of ninety-three feet. Early in the seventeenth century, the existing lines of water pipes were supplemented by a scheme devised by Edmund Colthurst and undertaken by Hugh Myddelton, which involved the construction of a channel, the New River, from Amwell and Chadwell in Hertfordshire to Clerkenwell, which was reached in 1613. From the New River Head, there, water was distributed around the city in elm pipes.

Whatever the dangers that the crowding and dirtiness of London were thought to pose, neither they nor the threat of plague deterred those arriving from elsewhere. Perhaps they were partly reassured by the preventatives and cures that were available. The College of Physicians' *Pharmacopoeia Londinensis* had been issued in 1618, with a second, enlarged, edition following soon afterwards, but both were in Latin and so of little use to lay people. With the collapse of controls on the press in the early 1640s, the numbers of titles published increased enormously during the 1640s and 1650s and the College lost control over publications on medical matters. In 1649, Nicholas Culpeper issued *A Physical Directory*, which was not only a translation into English of the College's *Pharmacopoeia*, but included 'many hundred additions' that it had not approved. Three years later, he followed this with *The English Physitian*, which, as *Culpeper's Complete Herbal*, was to become a best-seller. It offered 'a Compleat Method of Physick, whereby a man may preserve his Body in Health; or cure himself, being sick', using herbs which grew in England, with recommendations for the preparation of medicines.

These books undermined the College's attempts to control the practice of medicine and made information on plague remedies widely available to literate Londoners. For example, *angelica* was recommended by Culpeper because it 'resists Poison, by defending and comforting the Heart, Blood, and Spirits, it doth the like against the Plague, and all Epidemical Diseases if the Root be taken in powder to the weight of half a dram at a time with some good Treacle in Cardus Water, and the party thereupon laid to sweat in his Bed'. And its stalk and roots could be chewed as 'good preservatives in time of infection'. Many antidotes and treatments were already known and used, supplied by physicians or apothecaries, or by those condemned as quacks because they were unlearned and unqualified to practise medicine. But the availability of Culpeper's collections in print may have given further encouragement to those who remained fearful of the disease, despite its decline in the 1650s.

Those who were aware of the experience of other European cities during the decade would have been glad of the advice on preventatives which Culpeper included. Leiden provided a parallel with London in having grown rapidly since the late sixteenth century, and it again suffered severely from plague in 1654 and 1655, with more than 22,000 deaths in a population of roughly 60,000, its worst outbreak of the century; Amsterdam lost more than 16,000 of its citizens in 1655. The outbreak at Rotterdam in that year was less severe, producing a death rate of perhaps half that at Amsterdam, but plague erupted in many other north European ports during the middle years of the decade, including Bremen, Hamburg, Copenhagen and Danzig, and as far afield as central Russia, with an epidemic in Moscow in 1654. The response was to reconsider and improve existing arrangements. At Leiden, the wooden pesthouse built in 1635 was replaced by a brick building that resembled an almshouse rather than a short-term hospital.

In the western Mediterranean, Spain experienced outbreaks of plague between 1647 and 1652, with terrible epidemics in Seville in 1649 and Barcelona in 1651. The chronicler of the calamity at Seville, Diego Ortiz de Zunyiga, wrote that the city 'suffered a huge loss of inhabitants and next to nobody was left. A large number of dwellings lie empty, surely to become ruins in the years to come.' Some cities in Italy succumbed to the disease during the mid-1650s. Loss of life in Naples and Genoa in 1656–57 was proportionately higher than at Leiden, with more than fifty per cent of their citizens dying during plague epidemics, and Rome lost roughly twenty per cent of its population in those years. Father Antero Maria di San Bonaventura supervised operations in the Genoa pesthouse and survived to write an account of the experience, in which he questioned whether the city would have suffered any worse than it actually did if no measures had been taken against the disease. Doctors protected themselves from plague by wearing a waxen robe that covered the entire body and a mask that incorporated a beak filled with herbs, an outfit developed by French practitioners and adopted by their Italian counterparts.

Across much of Europe, these were the worst outbreaks since the 1630s, yet London escaped unscathed. In September 1655, the Council of State discussed with the Lord Mayor the steps which should be taken to prevent plague spreading from the Netherlands. It then put in place the quarantining of shipping, similar to the measures adopted earlier in the century. All those on board ships arriving at any English port had to identify themselves and their port of origin, and those from the Netherlands were to be held in quarantine for twenty days. If no plague symptoms appeared, the crews and passengers could land, but only in clothes brought from shore, because fabrics were thought to harbour the disease, and the cargoes were to be kept on board until further order.

Because of the implementation of the Council's policy, and chance factors beyond its control or understanding, London escaped the epidemics of the 1650s, which, as in the 1610s, broke the pattern that had so often seen it suffer in the wake of outbreaks of plague in the Low Countries. By the early 1660s, it had been free from a serious outbreak since 1636 and from a major epidemic since 1625, and even the increased risks of the war years in the 1640s had not produced a widespread plague epidemic in the capital. Astrologers such as William Lilly and Thomas Reeve continued to make mournful predictions of a dreadful pestilence to come, but the publication by Graunt of the figures from the Bills of Mortality illustrated the extent of the decline in the number of plague deaths.

Even those who were fearful that a change of reign would be quickly followed by an epidemic should have been reassured, because, as Graunt pointed out, although that had occurred at the accession of James I and Charles I, the pattern had not been repeated either in 1649, when Charles II nominally replaced his father, or 1660, when he effectively came to the throne. But uncertainty remained about the nature of the disease and the reasons for its dissemination. And so some aspects of the policy devised during the past 100 years or so were still not completely accepted as necessary or helpful, either by those who had experienced them or by the theorists. Without the co-operation of the population, that policy could not be entirely effective, and it was about to be put to a very tough test indeed.

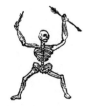

5

The Great Plague

The Levant was widely regarded as the source of plague and, because of the dominance of the Dutch in the carrying trade, the ports of Holland and Zeeland were thought to be the most likely places from which it was diffused around northern Europe. Direct English trade with the Mediterranean was also expanding during the mid-seventeenth century, exemplified by the doubling of cloth exports to the Ottoman empire between the 1620s and the early 1660s. And so the epidemic which erupted in Turkey in 1661 was a potential danger to London, magnified when the disease appeared at Amsterdam in 1663, gradually spreading throughout the United Provinces, and then at Hamburg.

Dutch physicians believed that the infection had reached Amsterdam from Algiers, not directly from Turkey, and Henry Oldenburg, the Secretary of the Royal Society, was confident that its progress could be traced, 'step by step'. Clearly, he had faith in the reliability of the recording of plague deaths across Europe. Nathaniel Hodges, on the other hand, thought that the plague had spread to Holland from Smyrna, on Turkey's Aegean coast. Whatever the source of the disease, the Privy Council was sufficiently alarmed in the autumn of 1663 to once again ask the Lord Mayor and aldermen for advice. They replied not with reference to previous practice, but 'after the example of other countries', and recommended that all vessels from the infected areas should be stopped from reaching London. Gravesend was designated as the furthest point upstream that suspect ships, both English and foreign, were to be allowed. Here some lazarettos should be provided, where the cargoes would be unloaded and aired for forty days, but with all members of the crew and passengers kept on board for the same period. At a meeting on 23 October, the Council accepted the recommendations, although two weeks later it referred the matter to a committee for further consideration.

The committee's report developed the policy of naval quarantine by suggesting that two Royal Navy ships should anchor as far down the Thames estuary as they could do with safety, to intercept shipping. Any vessels from places that were free from plague were to be issued with health certificates, but those from Amsterdam, Hamburg or any infected place would be asked to turn back. If they chose to continue their voyage, they had to serve a *trientane* of thirty days. Perhaps because of the difficulties of enforcement encountered by the customs officers when this policy had been employed earlier, they would be held not as far up the river as Gravesend, which was easily reached by the London watermen, but a further ten miles downstream, at

Hole Haven on Canvey Island. The island had been reclaimed around 1620 by Dutch engineers and had then been settled by Dutch labourers. Its remoteness made it a suitably secure place for a quarantine station. A Navy ketch, manned by six men, should cruise off the island when any vessels were in quarantine to prevent anyone slipping away from them prematurely, in a small boat. Any ships which evaded the naval cordon would be stopped by the garrisons at Tilbury fort on the north bank and the blockhouse at Gravesend on the opposite shore. This system of a double cordon was more sophisticated than the procedures which had been tried hitherto.

The new arrangements were in place by the middle of November, when three merchantmen and one warship were being held at Hole Haven. They had come from Holland and, although no one on board had developed any plague symptoms, the Council ordered that they should be detained for a further two weeks before being boarded and inspected. On 11 November, the Council extended 'the Method observed here in the River of Thames' to all ports, with the order that the period of isolation should be thirty days. In January it received a request for advice from Great Yarmouth, where the bailiffs were concerned about the risk from vessels arriving there from Amsterdam, and it repeated its earlier advice. The Council displayed some flexibility in releasing perishable cargoes of cod and peas, but they had to be brought upstream in other vessels, and that concession was not extended to the crews or passengers.

The spring of 1664 brought news that the epidemic in Holland was worsening, which prompted the Council to review its policy. Because Amsterdam had a regular trade with the other Dutch ports, all ships from the United Provinces were to be held at Hole Haven, and in May the Council ordered that the full forty-day period of quarantine should be observed. If anyone had come ashore from a vessel from the

United Provinces without serving the whole quarantine, the justices were to close the house where they were living for forty days, as if it contained someone with the plague. Such tightening of the restrictions was prompted by the growing epidemic on the continent and 'the heat of weather approaching, which renders the contagion more dangerous'. In July, the orders were extended to shipping from Hamburg, where the disease had broken out again.

The regulations 'to prevent the bringing in the Pest from the parts beyond the sea' were enforced so effectively that at the end of July, the Dutch ambassador protested that the trade of both countries was being adversely affected, to which the Council responded that Charles II was sympathetic to his appeal, but he had to protect his people from plague, 'which cannot be done without such restraints'. Rather than ease the restrictions, the Council tightened them further on 31 August, with an order that no people or goods were to be permitted to land at any port for the following three months, excepting only those ships which were already at sea. This drastic widening of the policy may have been designed to prevent any vessels gaining exemption by claiming to have come from a plague-free port, as well as an awareness that the epidemic in Holland had worsened. In May 1664, the number of deaths registered in Amsterdam was 338 in one week, and the figure had doubled by the end of July, when Sir George Downing reported to the Earl of Clarendon, the Lord Chancellor, that 'the plague is scattered generally over the whole country even in the little dorps and villages, and it is gott to Antwerp and Brussels'. The peak was 1,050 in a week and the weekly figure was 800, even at the end of September.

Britain's diplomatic relations with the United Provinces were becoming increasingly difficult and the quarantine regulations were a relatively minor issue. The smouldering rivalry between the two countries over trade was being fanned by

44 The reigns of James I and his son Charles I both began with major plague epidemics in London. They are depicted here in 1623; the jubilant Londoners in the background are celebrating the failure of negotiations for Charles to marry the King of Spain's sister.

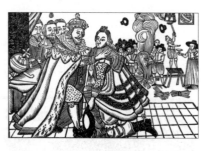

45 Death stands triumphantly on the coffins of Londoners, some of whom are trying to leave, but are repelled by armed countrymen. St Paul's cathedral is the prominent building in the city beyond the ghastly scenes. This woodcut was used as the frontispiece of Thomas Dekker's *A Rod for Run-awayes* (1625) and John Taylor's *The Fearefull Summer* (1636).

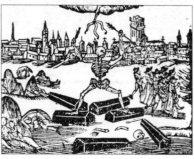

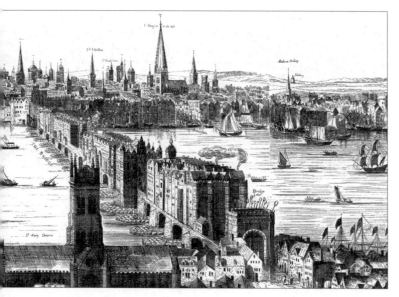

46 London Bridge in Visscher's *Panorama*, with Southwark in the foreground and the tall spire of the church of St Dunstan-in-the-East rising above the city. Nehemiah Wallington and his family lived throughout the plague epidemic of 1625 in their parish of St Leonard's, Eastcheap, just beyond the north end of the bridge.

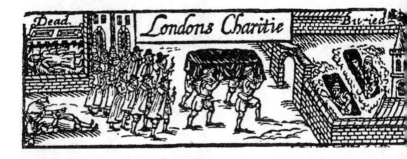

47 'London's Charitie' shows the orderly burial of the plague dead, with a coffin followed by mourners carrying sprigs of rosemary, and interments in individual graves. Despite official attempts to restrict the numbers attending a funeral, the citizens chose to continue their normal practices during epidemics.

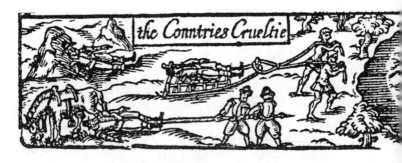

48 The bodies of those who died in the country were subject to much cruder handling, with uncovered bodies dragged on hurdles and deposited in a common grave. This broadsheet, *London's Lamentation* (1641), drew attention to the disquiet about the treatment meted out to those Londoners who left the city during epidemics.

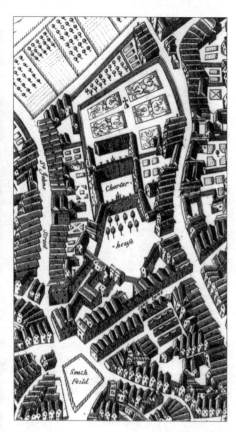

49 This section of Richard Newcourt's plan of London (1658) shows Smithfield and Clerkenwell, around the Charterhouse, where houses in one of the poorer neighbourhoods were described in 1635 as 'pore Raskoly habitations'.

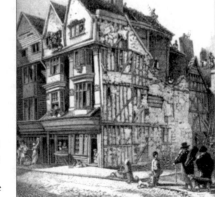

50 Seventeenth-century houses in Long Lane, Smithfield, which was a densely built-up district, with little or no space at the rear of the houses.

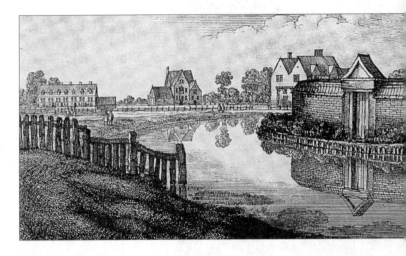

51 As London grew, new water supplies were provided, including the New River from Hertfordshire to Clerkenwell, which was completed in 1613. Wenceslaus Hollar's drawing shows a length of the New River in Islington.

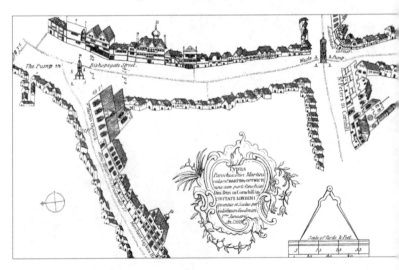

52 Plan of parts of the parishes of St Martin Outwich, to the left, and St Peter's, Cornhill, drawn in 1599. Both churches are shown, as is the line of the water pipes and the pumps at the junctions of Bishopsgate Street with Threadneedle Street (containing the Merchant Taylors' hall) and Leadenhall Street.

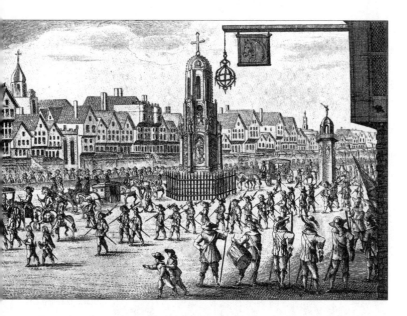

53 The procession bringing Charles I's mother-in-law, Marie de Medici, to London in 1638, escorted by members of London's militia, the Trained Bands, here passing the cross in Cheapside, its status as one of the wealthiest streets in the city shown by the large houses. The illustration is from Jean Puget de La Serre's *Entrée Royalle de la reyne mere du roy tres-Chrestien dans la ville de Londres* (1638).

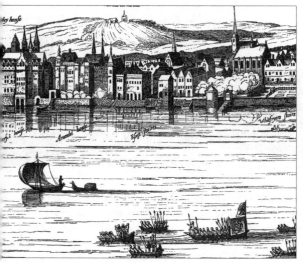

54 The riverfront running eastwards from the Savoy to the Temple, with its gardens. A resident of this area, who lived close to the Savoy, was a critical observer of the behaviour of Londoners during the plague in 1636.

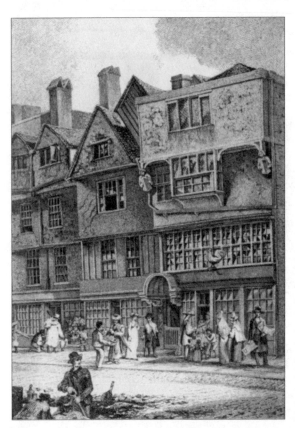

55 Four-storey houses in Leadenhall Street, with jettied upper floors overhanging the street, characteristic of the 'mishapen and extravagant Houses' complained of by the diarist John Evelyn.

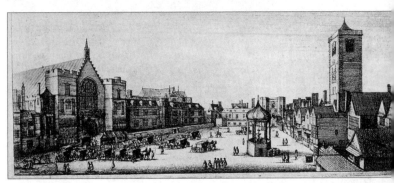

56 New Palace Yard, with Westminster Hall and the Clock House, an engraving by Wenceslaus Hollar, 1647. Fearful of the plague, in 1641 the House of Lords ordered that Members' coaches should wait only in New Palace Yard, to reduce possible contacts with plague in the areas nearby.

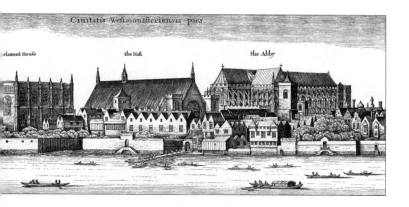

rlament Houſe   the Hall   the Abby

57 Westminster from the river, by Hollar, 1647. The conflict between Charles I and Parliament led to the the Civil War, bringing an increased risk of plague to London, which was at the centre of Parliament's war effort.

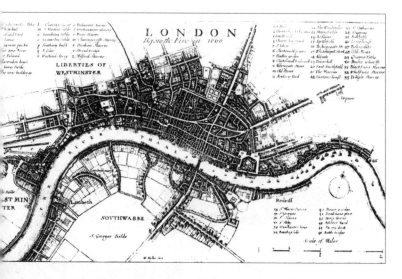

58 Hollar's plan of mid-seventeenth-century London shows the extent to which the city had expanded, both to the east, towards Stepney and along the river, and the west, where the West End was beginning to develop. Building along the riverside on the south bank stretched from Rotherhithe (Redriff) in the east almost to Lambeth.

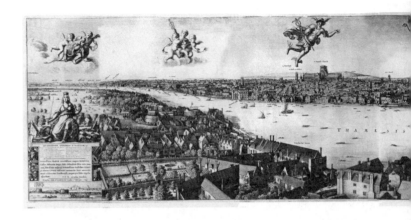

Above: 59 Hollar's Long View of London from Southwark, 1647, depicts a city which had grown to be the second largest in northern Europe, after Paris. Hollar conveys the density of the buildings on both sides of the river and the amount of seagoing shipping downstream from London Bridge.

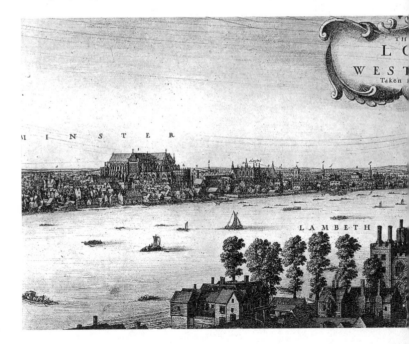

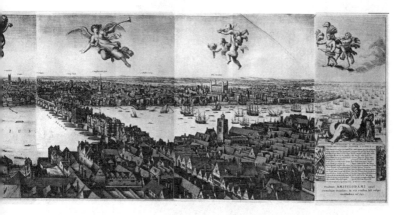

Below: 60 Hollar chose a different perspective in this later view across the Thames from Lambeth, which has Lambeth Palace in the foreground and the long sweep of the north side of the river from Westminster to St Paul's.

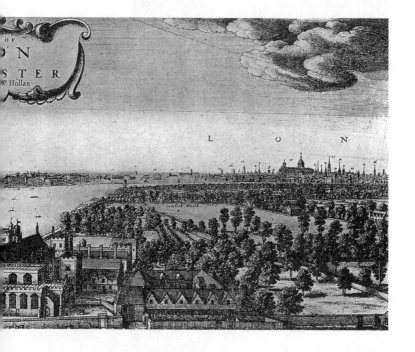

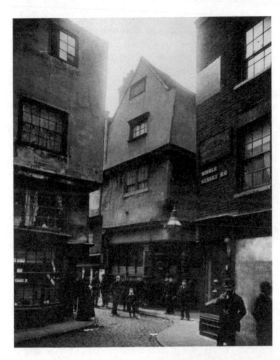

61 The narrow streets
and tall buildings
around Smithfield
c.1900, one of the
densely populated
parts of London
that suffered high
mortality during the
Great Plague of 1665.

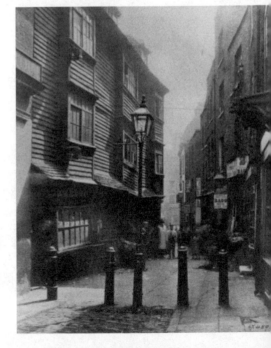

62 Peter's Lane,
Clerkenwell, c.1900,
on the north side of
Smithfield. The parish
of St James, Clerkenwell,
recorded almost six
times the annual average
number of deaths during
the Great Plague.

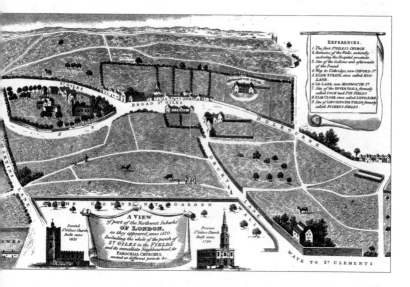

63 The parish of St Giles-in-the-Fields in 1570. The plague deaths recorded there in the early months of 1665 marked the beginning of the Great Plague and the parish was blamed, for not having effectively enforced household quarantine.

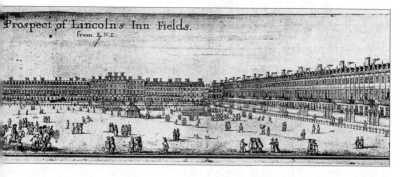

64 St Giles-in-the-Fields was in an area with much poor housing, but also wealthy neighbourhoods, such as Lincoln's Inn Fields, developed in the late 1630s and shown here on Hollar's engraving of c.1657.

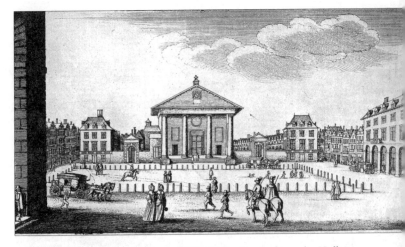

65 The Piazza in Covent Garden, with St Paul's church, drawn by Hollar. This was the wealthiest district in London in the mid-1660s and although it experienced a threefold increase in burials during the Great Plague, this was a relatively small rise compared with the poorer areas.

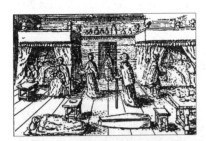

66 The Great Plague: the disease has struck this relatively well-to-do family, with the sick being nursed in their beds and a member of the household laid on the floor, close to a coffin.

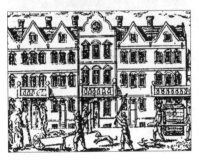

67 This street scene illustrates many of the aspects of a plague epidemic. The sedan-chair is for moving the sick to the pesthouse; the figure in the centre is a dog killer, taking aim at his victim, with a dead dog lying behind; the man wheeling the barrow is a scavenger; those carrying long rods are the searchers; and houses in the background have been closed, with crosses on their doors.

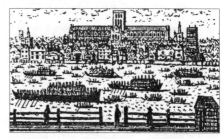

68 London's citizens flee from the city during the Great Plague, crowded into boats, which are being rowed past St Paul's.

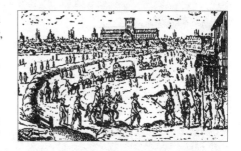

69 Londoners also leave by coach and wagon, on horse and on foot, streaming away from the city, with St Paul's in the background. They are met by hostile armed countrymen, to whom a citizen shows his health certificate for inspection. In the left foreground is the body of a plague victim.

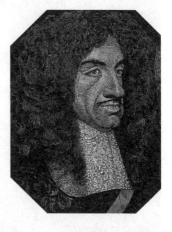

Right: 70 Charles II left Whitehall Palace at the end of June 1665 to accompany his mother, Henrietta Maria, to Dover. The court moved to Salisbury, then to Oxford, where the king summoned Parliament to meet in October.

Below: 71 The monarch was held to have the power to heal scrofula (the King's Evil) by touch, but because of plague the numbers of people coming close to the king had to be restricted for his safety, and so this advertisement was placed in *The Intelligencer* announcing that the practice was to be suspended.

This is to give notice, That His Majesty hath declared his positive resolution not to *heal* any more after the end of this present *April* until *Michaelmas* next : And this is published to the end that all Persons concerned may take notice thereof, and not receive a disappointment.

London, April 22.

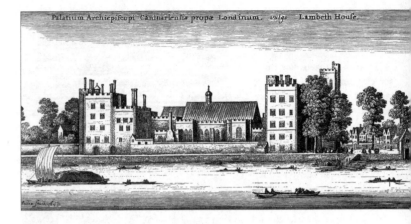

72 Lambeth Palace c.1647, by Hollar. This is the London residence of the Archbishop
Canterbury, where Archbishop Gilbert Sheldon remained during the Great Plague, se
reports to the court.

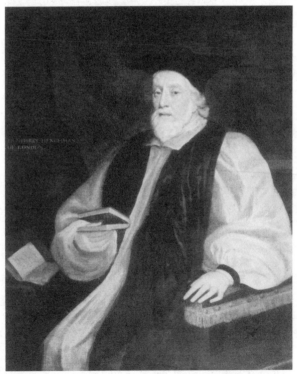

73 Humphrey
Henchman,
Bishop of
London,
remained in
the city and
warned those
parish clergy
who had left
that they would
be replaced if
they did not
return to their
duties.

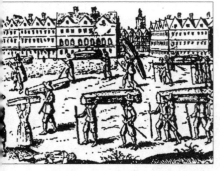

74 Bodies of plague victims being taken to burial during the Great Plague, mostly in coffins, although one is on a stretcher and another lies unattended to. The illustration shows that the victims were of all ages, for some coffins are carried by two or four men, but others, which must contain the bodies of children and infants, by just one man and a woman carries a small coffin above her head.

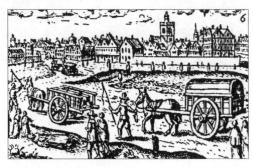

75 The increasing number of victims required the opening of large burial pits, to which bodies were taken on carts.

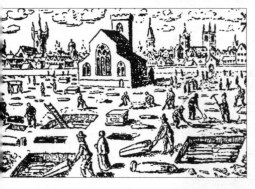

76 A busy burial scene during the Great Plague, perhaps at Cripplegate, with corpses in coffins and shrouds awaiting interment in neat rectangular pits, which are dug and refilled by numerous grave diggers.

77 A long procession follows a coffin to the grave, despite the order that only family members, not friends or neighbours, should attend funerals. The covering of the coffin and the dress of the mourners suggests that a wealthy or prominent citizen is being buried.

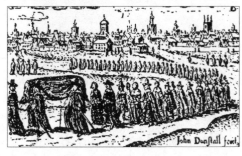

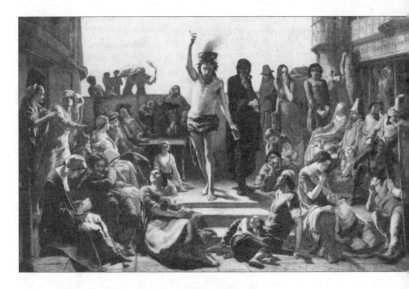

78 In his *A Journal of the Plague Year* (1722), Daniel Defoe mentions that 'the famous Solomon Eagle an Enthusiast... went about denouncing of Judgment upon the City in a frightful manner; sometimes quite naked, and with a Pan of burning Charcoal on his Head'. He based this anecdote on the behaviour of Solomon Eccles, a Quaker, who in the early 1660s had run naked through Bartholomew Fair with a pan of burning charcoal on his head, representing fire and brimstone, calling on London to repent. He was arrested in May 1665 and held in prison for several weeks.

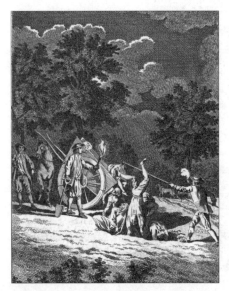

79 Samuel Wale's imaginative depiction of burials at Holywell Mount, Shoreditch, with the bodies, in neither shrouds nor coffins, dragged by a pole into a pit. Burials were indeed conducted at night and pipes were smoked in the belief that tobacco warded off the plague.

	Bur.	Plag.		Bur.	Plag.		Bur.	Plag.
St Alban Woodstreet	11	8	St George Botolphlane			St Martin Ludgate	4	4
Alhallows Barking	13	11	St Gregory by St Pauls	9	5	St Martin Organs	8	6
Alhallows Breadstreet	1	1	St Hellen	11	11	St Martin Outwitch	1	
Alhallows Great	6	5	St James Dukes place	7	5	St Martin Vintrey	17	17
Alhallows Honylane			St James Garlickhithe	3		St Matthew Fridaystreet	2	
Alhallows Lesse	3	2	St John Baptist	7	4	St Maudlin Milkstreet	2	2
Alhallows Lumbardstreet	6	4	St John Evangelist			St Maudlin Oldfishstreet	8	4
Alhallows Staining	7	5	St John Zachary	1	1	St Michael Bassishaw	12	11
Alhallows the Wall	23	11	St Katharine Coleman	5	1	St Michael Cornhil	3	
St Alphage	18	10	St Katharine Crechurch	7	4	St Michael Crookedlane	7	1
St Andrew Hubbard	1		St Lawrence Jewry	2	1	St Michael Queenhithe	4	6
St Andrew Undershaft	14	9	St Lawrence Pountney	6	5	St Michael Quern	1	
St Andrew Wardrobe	21	16	St Leonard Eastcheap	1		St Michael Royal	2	1
St Ann Aldersgate	18	11	St Leonard Fosterlane	17	13	St Michael Woodstreet	2	1
St Ann Blackfryers	22	17	St Magnus Parish	2	2	St Mildred Breadstreet	2	1
St Antholins Parish			St Margaret Lothbury	2	1	St Mildred Poultrey	4	3
St Austins Parish			St Margaret Moses			St Nicholas Acons		
St BartholomewExchange	2	2	St MargaretNewfishstreet	1		St Nicholas Coleabby	1	
St Bennet Fynck	2	2	St Margaret Pattons	1		St Nicholas Olaves	3	1
St Bennet Gracechurch			St Mary Abchurch	1		St Olave Hartstreet	7	4
St Bennet Paulswharf	16	8	St Mary Aldermanbury	11	5	St Olave Jewry	1	1
St Bennet Sherehog			St Mary Aldermary	2		St Olave Silverstreet	23	20
St Botolph Billingsgate	2		St Mary le Bow	6	6	St Pancras Soperlane		
Chrifts Church	27	22	St Mary Bothaw	1	1	St Peter Cheap	1	1
St Christophers	1		St Mary Colechurch			St Peter Cornhil	7	6
St Clement Eastcheap	2	2	St Mary Hill	2	1	St Peter Paulswharf	5	2
St Dionis Backchurch	2	1	St Mary Mounthaw	1		St Peter Poor	3	2
St Dunstan East	7	2	St Mary Sommerset	6	5	St Steven Colemanstreet	15	11
St Edmund Lumbardstr.	2	2	St Mary Stayning	1		St Steven Walbrook		
St Ethelborough	13	7	St Mary Woolchurch	1		St Swithin	2	2
St Faith	6	6	St Mary Woolnoth	1	1	St Thomas Apostle	8	7
St Foster	13	11	St Martin Iremongerlane			Trinity Parish	5	3
St Gabriel Fenchurch	1							

Christned in the 97 Parishes within the Walls — 34   Buried — 538   Plague — 366

	Bur.	Plag.		Bur.	Plag.		Bur.	Plag.
St Andrew Holborn	432	220	St Botolph Aldgate	238	212	Saviours Southwark	160	120
St Bartholomew Great	58	50	St Botolph Bishopsgate	288	236	S. Sepulchres Parish	403	274
St Bartholomew Lesse	19	15	St Dunstan West	36	29	St Thomas Southwark	24	21
St Bridget	147	119	St George Southwark	80	60	Trinity Minories	8	5
Bridewel Precinct	7	5	St Giles Cripplegate	847	572	At the Pesthouse	9	9
St Botolph Aldersgate	70	61	St Olave Southwark	235	131			

Christned in the 16 Parishes without the Walls — 61   Buried, and at the Pesthouse — 2861   Plague — 2139

	Bur.	Plag.		Bur.	Plag.		Bur.	Plag.
St Giles in the fields	204	175	Lambeth Parish	13	9	St Mary Islington	50	45
Hackney Parish	12	8	St Leonard Shoreditch	252	168	St Mary Whitechappel	319	270
St James Clerkenwel	172	172	St Magdalen Bermondsey	57	36	Rotherith Parish	7	2
St Kath. near the Tower	40	34	St Mary Newington	74	52	Stepney Parish	371	273

Christned in the 12 out Parishes in Middlesex and Surry — 49   Buried — 1571   Plague — 1244

	Bur.	Plag.		Bur.	Plag.		Bur.	Plag.
St Clement Danes	94	78	St Martin in the fields	255	193	St Margaret Westminster	220	191
St Paul Covent Garden	18	16	St Mary Savoy	11	10	Whereof at the Pesthouse		13

Christned in the 5 Parishes in the City and Liberties of Westminster — 27   Buried — 598   Plague — 488

80 The Bill of Mortality for the third week of August 1665 shows relatively small numbers of plague deaths in the central parishes, compared to those in the parishes around the walls and in the suburbs.

The Diseases and Casualties this Week.

Abortive	4	Imposthume	8
Aged	45	Infants	22
Bleeding	1	Kingsevil	4
Broken legge	1	Lethargy	1
Broke her scull by a fall in the street at St. Mary VVool-church	1	Livergrown	1
		Meagrome	1
		Palsie	1
Childbed	28	Plague	4237
Chrisomes	9	Purples	2
Consumption	126	Quinsie	5
Convulsion	89	Rickets	23
Cough	1	Riting of the Lights	18
Dropsie	53	Rupture	1
Feaver	348	Scurvy	3
Flox and Small-pox	11	Shingles	1
Flux	1	Spotted Feaver	166
Frighted	2	Stilborn	4
Gowt	1	Stone	2
Grief	3	Stopping of the stomach	17
Griping in the Guts	79	Strangury	3
Head-mould-shot	1	Suddenly	2
Jaundies	7	Surfeit	74
		Teeth	111
		Thrush	6
		Tissick	9
		Ulcer	1
		Vomiting	10
		Winde	4
		Wormes	20

Christned { Males — 90 / Females — 81 / In all — 171 }	Buried { Males — 2777 / Females — 2791 / In all — 5568 }	Plague — 4237

Increased in the Burials this Week ——————— 249
Parishes clear of the Plague ——— 27   Parishes Infected ——— 103

The Assize of Bread set forth by Order of the Lord Maior and Cours of Aldermen,
A penny Wheaten Loaf to contain Nine Ounces and a half, and three
half-penny White Loaves the like weight.

81 The reverse of that Bill provides the totals for the causes of death, with 4,237 of the total of 5,568 attributed to plague.

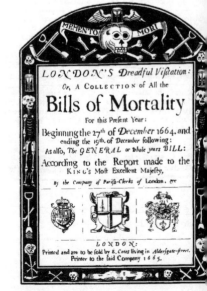

82 The figures for the year were published in a collection and summary of the Bills of Mortality, expressively entitled *London's Dreadful Visitation.*

A generall Bill for this present year,

ending the 19 of *December* 1665 according to the Report made to the KINGS most Excellent Majesty.

By the Company of Parish Clerks of London, &c.

Parish	Buried	Plag.	Parish	Buried	Plag.	Parish	Buried	Plag.	Parish	Buried	Plag.
St Albans Woodstreet	200	121	St Clements Eastcheap	28	20	St Margaret Moses	38	25	St Michael Cornehill	164	52
St Alhallowes Barking	514		St Dionis Back-church	78	27	St Margat New Fishst.	114	66	St Michael Crookedla.	179	132
St Alhallowes Breadst.	35	16	St Dunstans East	265	150	St Margaret Pattons	49	24	St Michael Queenhith	203	122
St Alhallowes Great	455	426	St Edmunds Lumbard	70	36	St Mary Abchurch	99	54	St Michael Queene	44	18
St Alhallowes Honi-lane			St Ethelborough	105	106	St Mary Aldermanbury	181	109	St Michael Royall	116	116
St Alhallowes Lesse	230	175	St Faiths	104	70	St Mary Aldermary	105	75	St Michael Woodstreet	122	62
St Alhall. Lumbardst.	90	62	St Fosters	144	105	St Mary le Bow	64	30	St Mildred Breadstreet	59	26
St Alhall. Stayning	185		St Gabriel Fen-church	69	39	St Mary Bothaw	55	30	St Mildred Poultrey	68	46
St Alhall. westthe Wall	500		St George Botolphlane	41	27	St Mary Colechurch	17	8	St Nicholas Acons	46	33
St Alphage	271		St Gregories by Paules	376	232	St Mary Hill	94	64	St Nicholas Coleabby	125	91
St Andrew Hubbard	71	25	St Hellens	108	75	St Mary Mounthaw	56	37	St Nicholas Olaver	90	62
St Andrew Vndershaft	274	189	St James Dukes place	262	190	St Mary Summerset	342	262	St Olaves Hart-streete	237	150
St Andrew Wardrobe	476	309	St James Garlickhithe	189	118	St Mary Stainings	47	27	St Olaves Jewry	54	32
St Anne Aldersgate	282	197	St John Baptist	138	83	St Mary Woolchurch	65	33	St Olaves Silverstreet	250	132
St Anne Blacke-Friers	652	467	St John Euangelist	9		St Mary Woolnoth	75	38	St Pancras Soperlane	30	13
St Antholines Parish	58	33	St John Zacharie	85	54	St Martins Iremonger.	23		St Peters Cheape	115	62
St Austins Parish	45		St Katherine Coleman	299	213	St Martins Ludgate	196	128	St Peters Cornehill	136	76
St Barthol. Exchange	73	51	St Katherine Cree-chu	335	231	St Martins Organs	110	71	St Peters Paula Wharfe	114	86
St Bennet Fynch	23		St Lawrence Iewrie	94	48	St Martins Outwitch	60	34	St Peters Poore	79	47
St Bennet Grace-chu.	17		St Lawrence Pountney	214	140	St Martins Vintrey	417	349	St Stevens Colemanst	560	301
St Bennet Paul Wharf	355		St Leonard Eastcheape	42	17	St Matthw Fridayst.	24	6	St Stevens Walbrooke	34	17
St Bennet Sherehog	11		St Leonard Fosterlane	335	255	St Maudlins Milkstreet	44	22	St Swithins	93	56
St Botolph Billingsgate	111	60	St Magnus Parish	103	60	St Maudlin Oldfishstr.	176	121	St Thomas Apostle	163	110
Christ Church	653	467	St Margaret Lothbury	100	60	St Martins Vintrey	253	164	Trinitie Parish	115	79
St Christophers	60	47									

Buried in the 97 Parishes within the walls, — 15207   Whereof, of the Plague — 9887

Parish	Buried	Plag.	Parish	Buried	Plag.	Parish	Buried	Plag.
St Andrew Holborne	3958	3103	Bridewell Precinct —	230	179	St Dunstans Well.	958	665
St Bartholmew Great	493	344	St Botolph Aldersgate	997	755	St George Southwark	1613	1260
St Bartholmew Lesse	197	139	St Botolph Algate —	4926	4051	St Giles Cripplegate	8069	4838
St Bridget	2111	1427	St Botolph Bishopsgate	3464	2500	St Olaves Southwark	4793	2785

(and further entries, including St Saviours Southwark, Sepulchres Parish, Thomas Southwark, Trinity Minories, At the Pesthouse — 159, 156)

Buried in the 16 Parishes without the Walls — 41351   Whereof of the Plague — 28888

Parish	Buried	Plag.	Parish	Buried	Plag.
St Giles in the Fields	4457	3216	St Katherines Tower	956	601
Hackney Parish	132	132	Lambeth Parish	798	537
St James Clarkenwell	1803	1377	St Leonards Shoreditch	2669	1949

(St Magdalens Bermondsey 1943 1362; St Mary Newington 1272 1004; St Mary Islington 696 593; St Mary Whitechappel 4766 3855; Redriff Parish 304 210; Stepney Parish 8598 6583)

Buried in the 12 out-Parishes in Middlesex and Surrey — 28554   Whereof, of the Plague — 21420

Parish	Buried	Plag.	Parish	Buried	Plag.
St Clement Danes	1969	1319	St Mary Savoy	303	198
St Paul Covent Garden	408	261	St Margaret Westmin.	4710	3742
St Martins in the Fields	4804	3883	thereof at the Pesthouse	156	

Buried in the 5 Parishes in the City and Liberties of Westminster — 8403   Whereof of the Plague — 6203

The Total of all the Christnings —	9967
The Total of all the Burials this year —	97306
Whereof, of the Plague —	68596

Diseases and Casualties this year.

Disease	Count	Disease	Count	Disease	Count
Abortive and Stilborne	617	Executed	21	Palsie	30
Aged	1545	Flox and Smal Pox	655	Plague	68596
Ague and Feaver	5257	Found dead in streets, fields,&c.	20	Planet	6
Appoplex and Suddenly	116	Frighted	23	Plurisie	15
Bedrid	10	French Pox	86	Poysoned	1
Blasted	5	Gout and Sciatica	27	Quinsie	35
Bleeding	16	Grief	46	Rickets	557
Bloudy Flux, Scowring & Flux	185	Griping in the Guts	1288	Rising of the Lights	397
Burnt and Scalded	8	Hang'd & made themselves away	7	Rupture	34
Calenture	3	Headmould shot & Mouldfallen	14	Scurvy	105
Cancer, Gangrene and Fistula	56	Jaundies	110	Shingles and Swine pox	2
Canker, and Thrush	111	Impostume	227	Sores, Ulcers, broken and bruised Limbes	82
Childbed	625	Kild by several accidents	46	Spleen	14
Chrisomes and Infants	1258	Kings Evill	86	Spotted Feaver and Purples	1929
Cold and Cough	68	Leprosie	2	Stopping of the Stomach	332
Collick and Winde	134	Lethargy	14	Stone and Strangury	98
Consumption and Tissick	4808	Livergrowne	20	Surfet	1251
Convulsion and Mother	2036	Meagrom and Headach	12	Teeth and Worms	2614
Distracted	5	Measles	7	Vomiting	51
Dropsie and Timpany	1478	Murthered, and Shot	9	Wenn	1
Drowned	50	Overlaid and Starved	45		

Christened	Males — 5114; Females — 4853; In all — 9967
Buried	Males — 48569; Females — 48737; In all — 97306	Of the Plague — 68596

Increased in the Burials in the 130 Parishes and at the Pest-house this year — 79009
Increased in the Plague in the 130 Parishes and at the Pest-house this year — 68590

FACSIMILE REPRODUCTION OF A GENERAL BILL FOR THE YEAR 1665 IN POSSESSION OF THE AUTHOR

83 The summary of the Bills for 1665 shows the numbers buried and those deaths attributed to plague, by parish, and the total numbers by cause of death. The number buried was almost ten times the number of babies christened.

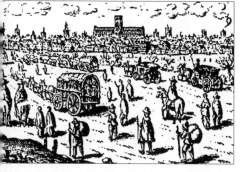

84 As the number of plague deaths recorded in the Bills declined, those who had left London steadily returned to the city.

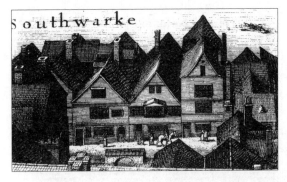

Left: 85 Southwark suffered badly in the Great Plague; the crowded buildings there were shown on Hollar's engraving of 1647.

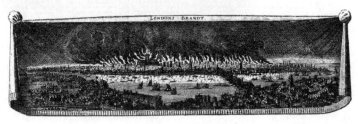

Above: 86 The Great Plague was followed in September 1666 by the Great Fire of London, which destroyed 13,200 houses, 87 churches and the halls of 44 of the livery companies, and attracted horrified attention across Europe. This is a German print of the disaster.

Left: 87 The title page of *A Journal of the Plague Year* by Daniel Defoe. Published in 1722, this fictional account was based on authentic sources from 1665 and has had an enduring influence on posterity's perception of the Great Plague in London.

A
JOURNAL
OF THE
𝔓lague 𝔜ear:
BEING
Obſervations or Memorials,
Of the moſt Remarkable
OCCURRENCES,
As well
PUBLICK *as* PRIVATE,
Which happened in
L O N D O N
During the laſt
GREAT VISITATION
In 1665.

Written by a CITIZEN who continued all the while in *London*. Never made publick before

L O N D O N:
Printed for *E. Nutt* at the *Royal-Exchange*; *J. Roberts* in *Warwick-Lane*; *A. Dodd* without *Temple-Bar*; and *J. Graves* in St. *James's-ſtreet*. 1722.

aggressive actions instigated by a coterie at court that centred around James, Duke of York. In 1664, a British flotilla under Sir Robert Holmes cruised around the coast of west Africa, capturing the Dutch trading posts and intercepting their shipping. The Dutch retaliated by sending a fleet under Michiel de Ruyter to reverse these British successes. Arriving off Gorée on 11 October, within a few weeks he had done just that, leaving only Cape Coast Castle in British hands. But even earlier, in late July, Samuel Pepys, Clerk of the Acts to the Navy Board, had noted in his diary that 'All our discourse is of a Dutch war; and I find it is likely to come to it.'

After the campaigns by Holmes and de Ruyter, war became ever more probable, and the Council made an order on 28 October that all ships should be forbidden to leave any port in England and Wales. The only exceptions were those engaged in internal trade between British ports, the East India Company's vessels and those which were carrying fish for export. This limited the opportunities for the capture of British ships, should the Dutch begin commerce raiding before a declaration of war. The Council rescinded the order at the end of November, except for Dutch ships, but re-imposed it in mid-December for all vessels. Such a reduction in sailings, at least to European destinations, had the benefit of keeping available as many sailors as possible for manning His Majesty's ships. The fleet had a complement of 16,000, but needed 30,000 if it was to be put on a war footing. For their part, the Dutch took a similar step by ordering their ships not to enter British ports, in case of seizure, and so trade between Britain and the United Provinces should have come to a virtual standstill. So far as protection against the transmission of plague was concerned, this was ideal.

The epidemic at Amsterdam had declined during the winter, although there were 24,148 deaths in the city during 1664, in a population approaching 200,000 before the outbreak. In

London, there were only five recorded plague deaths during the year. The metropolis had virtually escaped infection, either from abroad or from Great Yarmouth, where the disease had broken out during the autumn. As in 1655, in similar circumstances, this seemed to vindicate the policy of quarantining shipping, which could be justified by the other benefits that it produced. It made customs evasion more difficult, allowed imports to be regulated, provided information on what goods were in port, so that they could be released on to the market when necessary, and allowed checks to be kept on who was entering the country and for what purpose – whether they were merchants or travellers, for instance.

Satisfaction with the success of the policy in avoiding an outbreak in 1664 was high, because the weather had been so threatening. The summer was thundery, with heavy downpours, and William Boghurst, in St Giles-in-the-Fields, noted that:

...there was such a multitude of flyes that they lined the insides of houses, and if any threads or stringes did hang downe in any place, it was presently thicke sett with flyes like a rope of oniones, and swarms of Ants covered the highways that you might have taken up a handfull at a tyme, both winged and creeping Ants; and such a multitude of croaking froggs in ditches that you might have heard them before you saw them.

So the humid conditions associated with plague existed, and the ports in the Low Countries, so often the source of the disease, were experiencing a serious epidemic, yet London had escaped. But there was some cause for concern. In Boghurst's parish, smallpox had been the most common disease during the year, with about forty families contracting the disease, although he did admit that: 'The plague hath put itself forth in St. Giles', St. Clement's, St Paul's, Covent Garden, and St.

Martin's this 3 or 4 yeares, as I have been certainly informed by the people themselves that had it in their houses in those Parishes'. As an apothecary who was prepared to go into the homes of the sick to administer medicines, he was well placed to know, and his account is more dependable than the figures in the Bills.

During the winter, plague policy was a far less pressing issue for the Council than the deteriorating relations with the Dutch, who declared war on 22 February, undeterred by the effects of the epidemic. The declaration came too early in the year for operations to begin soon afterwards, in what was to be a purely naval war, especially as the winter was a cold one. The chilly weather also made it improbable that there would be many cases of plague before the spring. And the attention of the Privy Council, which met three times a week, was chiefly focused on the preparations for war. Pepys attended one of its committees that was discussing the impressment of seamen for the fleet, and was dismayed by the disorderliness of the meeting, noting that its members '...never sit down – one comes, now another goes, then comes another – one complaining that nothing is done, another swearing that he has been there these two hours and nobody came'. As they chatted, some of them praised 'the discipline of the late times', especially during the First Dutch War in the mid-1650s, and lamented that it had declined and drunkenness had increased, expressing their fears that 'our evil-living will call the hand of God upon us again'. Such a view of impending divine judgement for sin was to be expected from the Puritans and Presbyterians, now excluded from power, but it is more surprising to find it uttered by members of Charles II's government.

The Bills of Mortality recorded one plague death in the second week of February and two in the third week of April, and the Council turned its attention to the danger once more. On 26 April, aware that plague had broken out, or was 'vehemently suspected', in St Giles-in-the-Fields, it ordered the justices to inspect the houses containing suspected cases and close them if the disease was present, and to put the other customary regulations in place. These met with hostility. Within two days of the Council's order, the Sign of the Ship in that parish was closed on the justices' instructions and a cross and paper were attached to the door, only to be removed and the door opened 'in a riotous manner & the people of the house permitted, to goe abroad into the street promiscuously, with others'. This was an ominous beginning to the problem of enforcement. So far, the numbers of cases were small, but fear was growing, perhaps indicating the citizens' scepticism regarding the accuracy of the Bills in recording plague deaths. Pepys' summary of April concluded with the note that there were: 'Great fears of the Sickenesse here in the City, it being said that two or three houses are already shut up. God preserve us all.'

The Bill for the week ending 9 May included nine plague deaths, and the Council responded three days later by appointing a committee to consider the best way of preventing the spread of the disease, to implement both the former orders and any new ones that seemed appropriate. They ordered the Westminster justices, who were responsible for St Giles-in-the-Fields, to clear the pesthouse of those who were living there, so that plague cases could be moved into it, and authorised the setting of a rate to raise funds for building more pesthouses or 'other habitations'. As in earlier outbreaks, attention was given to the cleanliness of public places and the scouring of ditches. Householders were instructed to clean the street in front of their houses 'all the weeke long' and wash it down two or three times a day, and laystalls were to be moved if they were too close to thoroughfares.

Foul smells were to be prevented as far as possible and so putrid fish, bad corn, rotten fruit and hot bread were banned from sale, and old clothes were not to be sold. Stray pigs were to be impounded, no dogs, cats, rabbits and pigeons were to be kept within the city, and the dogs were to be killed by the designated dog-catchers. During the year, 353 dogs were killed in St Margaret's, Westminster and at least 4,380 in the City, with approximately 40,000 dogs and 200,000 cats slaughtered across London. Anyone in an official capacity who visited infected houses, such as physicians or examiners, was to carry a white rod, four feet long. The laws against inmates were to be enforced and the justices were to reduce the number of alehouses, but leaving enough to quarter the soldiers which the Duke of Albermarle thought necessary.

In the event, Albermarle did not billet his soldiers in the city, leaving a garrison in the Tower of London and moving the others to a tented encampment in Hyde Park. Neither detachment escaped the plague. The pesthouse for Tower Hamlets received fifty-eight soldiers from the Tower, and a pesthouse had to be built in Hyde Park to accommodate the sick. A soldier there produced a pamphlet, 'for the Information of such as were not Eye-Witnesses, of the Souldiers' sufferings'. They seem to have experienced some confusion as well as plague, losing or perhaps bartering many of their weapons, for a warrant issued in October 1666 required that 'two hundred matche lock muskets one hundred pikes and six score Collars of Bandaliers bee delivered... for the use of his Majesties Regiment of Guards in liew of armes lost by the said Regiment in the time of the Contagion of the pestilence'.

Within the city, the parishes should already have had designated examiners, watchmen, searchers and nurses. Surgeons were to be appointed to deal only with those suffering from the plague. Householders were required to give notice of suspected plague symptoms within two hours of their appearance and quarantine was to be served in the house, or in another house belonging to the householder. This tacitly gave approval to the movement of the sick from the building where they were taken ill, and they could also be moved to one of the pesthouses or, if they were full, to a hut or tent. The policy tried in 1625 and 1636, of transferring the sick to temporary encampments on the edge of the city, was again employed, with the direction that huts should be set up in Marylebone and on suitable sites elsewhere. Those who were to be removed were carried in coaches or sedan chairs, to limit their contact with others. As passengers could not be carried in coaches used for suspected plague victims, dedicated pest-coaches were employed. Someone who had been in contact with an infected person and was to be taken back to their parish to serve their quarantine was to be moved at night, and funerals were to take place during the hours of darkness, unattended by friends, neighbours or children. No coffins were to stand in a church during services and children were to be kept away from the corpse, coffin and grave.

The policies were the established ones and were put in place promptly, with the Council reacting more to the reports of plague than the hard evidence of recorded numbers in the Bills, which showed seventeen plague deaths in the last week of May. John Allin, who was studying physic, took a sceptical view of the returns in the Bills and thought that the true number of plague victims that week was three times the figure entered in them. The Council itself had become aware of plague deaths being certified as cases of 'spotted fever' by the searchers, and ordered its committee to investigate. Allin was living in Horsleydown, on the south side of the river, opposite the Tower, and commented that 'At the upper end of the towne persons high and low are very fearfull of it, and many removed'. Lady Sandwich was one of those who was 'afeared of the sickness and resolved to be gone into the country', yet she was not too fearful to stay a few days longer to see the outcome of a society elopement, in which she had a family interest.

In Covent Garden, Thomas Rugge's reaction was much more detached, for when he noted the sharp rise in the following week, with forty-three deaths from plague, he also commented that only five of the 130 parishes were infected. Rugge remarked that the playhouses were crowded with people during May, but they were closed on the Lord Chamberlain's order on 5 June. Two days later, Pepys noticed houses in Drury Lane marked with the regulation red cross and papers with the words 'Lord have mercy upon us'. Although he was thirty-two, this was the first time in his life that he had seen houses identified in this way and he was so alarmed for himself, and suddenly aware of his own smell, that he bought some tobacco to sniff and chew, 'which took away the apprehension'. He may have heard of its supposed preventative qualities in a tavern a fortnight earlier, when the conversation had turned to the news 'of the plague growing upon us in this town and of remedies against it; some saying one thing, some another'. According to Nathaniel Hodges, Londoners 'terrified each other with remembrances of a former pestilence; for it was a received notion amongst the common people, that the Plague visited England once in twenty years'. The last major epidemic had indeed been exactly forty years ago, in 1625, although the outbreaks in 1636 and the 1640s did not fit their chronology.

On 21 June, the Council attempted to contain the disease within St Giles by ordering the constables of the adjoining parishes to mount guard at the parish boundary and turn back vagrants, 'loose persons', or anyone suspected of coming from an infected house. This measure was surely imposed too late to be effective and in any case was impractical. Already, there were concerns that not enough men were willing to act as warders for such a task and to guard the houses that were closed. If the parishes found that they were short of warders, they were authorised to delegate the job to those who were drawing financial assistance from the parish funds, with the warning that if they refused they would lose their pensions. This draconian threat could have applied at this stage only in St Giles and the neighbouring districts, where the disease was most virulent. The weekly figures for plague deaths in the last three weeks of June were 112, 168 and 267, and fifty-eight per cent of the total for the month had been in St Giles, with just eighteen within the city walls.

Even so, the rising numbers of deaths during June were enough to convince Londoners that the outbreak would not subside, but would develop into a full-blown epidemic across the city as the weather became warmer. The beginning of the month had been unseasonably hot; Pepys thought that 7 June was the hottest day that he had ever experienced and noted that others described it as 'the hottest day they ever knew in England in the beginning of June'. Three days later, he was appalled to hear of a plague death at the house of his friend Dr Burnet in Fenchurch Street, not far from Seething Lane, where the Pepyses lived. On 17 June, he went to visit the Lord Treasurer, the Earl of Southampton, on business, only to find that he had left because of the danger. Pepys took a coach to return to the City, but going along Holborn he noticed that the coachman was driving slower and slower, and 'at last stood still, and came down hardly able to stand; and told me that he was suddenly stroke very sick and almost blind, he could not see'. Pepys thought that this had been his first contact with the disease, which 'stroke me very deep', yet he was not afraid to transfer to another coach, and at this time he still travelled by coach or took a wherry on the river. At Cripplegate, a few days later, he noticed the numbers leaving London, with 'the coaches and waggons being all full of people going into the country', and his own impression that the plague 'increases mightily' was reinforced by the sight of a closed house opposite

St Clement's church, significant because it stood 'in the open street', not in an alley.

At the end of the month, the court broke up and left, going to Syon House and then Hampton Court, before moving on to Salisbury. When plague appeared there, it moved again, to Oxford, where Parliament assembled in October. Because the court went so far from the capital, regulations of the kind issued in 1636 to clear Londoners away from the vicinity of the royal palaces near London were not necessary. But, as Pepys had noticed, many wanted to leave the city, not just those dependent on the court, and they needed health certificates to allow them to pass the checks that were being set up to prevent those suspected of being infected entering a town or village. By early July, rumours were circulating of forged certificates, and so advertisements were placed by parish officers to give assurance that they would issue them only to those whom they really knew to be free from the disease, and that their certificates would be printed, not hand-written. The process cannot have long delayed the departure of those who were determined to leave. Nathaniel Hodges wrote almost scornfully when recounting 'with what precipitation the trembling inhabitants left the city, and how they flocked in such crowds out of town, as if London had quite gone out of itself, like the hurry of a sudden conflagration, all doors and passages are thronged for escape'.

Thomas Vincent had been rector of St Mary Magdalen, Milk Street, until he was ejected from the living in 1662 as a nonconformist, and he remained in London during the epidemic, as a critical observer of those who fled. He described the process in similar terms to those used by Benjamin Spencer forty years earlier: 'The great orbs begin first to move; the lords and gentry retire into their countries; their remote houses are prepared, goods removed, and London is quickly upon their backs.' After they had left, 'rich tradesmen provide themselves to depart; if they have not country-houses, they seek lodgings abroad for themselves and families, and the poorer tradesmen, that they may imitate the rich in their fear, stretch themselves to take a country journey, though they have scarce where-withal to bring them back again'. Pepys' mistress, Betty Martin, had left before the end of June. She was a linen-draper with a stall in Westminster Hall – her husband had a post in the Ordnance Office in the Tower – and could not have been described as wealthy, or comfortably off, and her departure supports Vincent's observation.

Among those who departed were some of the clergy, both parish ministers and senior clergymen. William Sancroft, installed as Dean of St Paul's in the previous December, went to Tunbridge Wells, where he had apparently been advised by his physician to go 'long before any plague was heard of'. Stephen Bing, a minor canon of St Paul's, kept him informed of developments in London. Towards the end of July, he distinguished between those minor canons and vicars of the cathedral who had left and those who 'only speake of going out of Towne', but a month later just three of the minor canons and two of the vicars remained.

Recorded deaths during July confirmed that those who had anticipated a major epidemic had been correct. The weekly numbers of deaths from plague rose from 470 to 2,010 during the month, and all deaths from 1,006 to 3,014. By the end of July, the disease had spread across much of London, to the extra-mural parishes on the north and north-east sides of the walls, to Southwark, and even into the City itself, where deaths were four times higher than the annual average for the previous ten years. Across London, the mortality rate was almost ten times higher than the ten-year average. The death toll continued to rise during August, when the number of infected parishes rose from eighty-six to 113, leaving only seventeen clear. And the successive weekly Bills returned 2,817, 3,880, 4,237 and 6,102 plague deaths. During July, there had been 8,828 deaths from all causes, sixty-four per cent of them attributed to plague; in August, the comparable figure was 22,413, with seventy-six per cent of them recorded as from plague.

As the danger increased, the reaction of Henry Oldenburg, who lived in Pall Mall, was that 'I strive to banish both fear and overconfidence, leading a regular life and avoiding the infected places as much as I can, leaving the rest to God and "neither fearing nor longing for my final hour"'. His was a prudent approach, yet with a touch of fatalism. Early in July, Pepys noticed houses in Pall Mall and the Piazza at Covent Garden shut up because of the plague, among many others across the city. He resolved to put his affairs in order, send his wife away to Woolwich for safety and finish all his business at the office during daylight, 'the season growing so sickly that it is much to be feared how a man can scape having a share with others in it'. His determination to finish work before dark was presumably because the burials of plague victims took place during the hours of darkness, yet he could not hold to his resolution, and just a few days later he travelled upriver to Mortlake to make a social visit and came back by boat, arriving home at two o'clock in the morning, regardless of the danger.

Pepys was not alone in being inconsistent – on the one hand, aware of the precautions he should take, while on the other continuing with some sort of normal life, flirting with young women, making social calls, and continuing to travel through London by coach and boat. Fear of going into company did not deter the citizens from attending church. On 27 July, Bing told Sancroft that 'People frequent the Church as before, excepting on Sundays, and the last Holyday', and on 3 August he wrote that 'we had on the Fast Day a laudable Sermon by Mr. Risden minister in Bread-street, my Lord Mayor being present, Sir Richard Brown and Sir John Robinson and other

Aldermen, with a great congregation'. Before Sancroft had left for Kent, Humphrey Henchman, Bishop of London, had asked him for copies of the forms of service issued in 1625, 1636 and 1640, to help them compile a new one. This was duly issued to the parishes, to be read on Wednesdays, the fast days for the plague, when worshippers should go to church 'and with penitent hearts to pray unto God to turn these Plagues from us, which we through our unthankfulness, and sinful lives have deserved'. The prayers included pleas for forgiveness 'for our iniquities and manifold transgressions', so that the plague should be ended, together with a practical request for 'Seasonable Weather, and good Air, and wholsom Food, and powerful Medicines, and whatever else thou seest to be good, and profitable for us'.

So far as the weather was concerned, it must have seemed that these prayers were answered, for, according to Hodges, 'the whole summer was refreshed with moderate breezes, sufficient to prevent the air's stagnation and corruption, and to carry off the pestilential streams; the heat was likewise too mild to encourage such corruption and fermentation as helps to taint the animal fluids, and prevent them from their natural state'. Boghurst's account supports this, with the observation that the plague was 'ushered in' with seven months of dry weather and westerly winds until July, although he also noted that when rain was followed by very hot weather 'the disease increased much', with the higher level of humidity. And so the pernicious, warm, southerly winds had not brought the plague, nor had the conditions been conducive to stagnant, foul air. Pondering the reasons for the spread of plague, Clarendon concluded that 'the ayre is not infected', although Simon Patrick, Rector of St Paul's, Covent Garden, attributed the large numbers of deaths in early September to the fact that the prevailing winds were then predominantly from the south, which were 'always observed to be bad in such Times'.

Professional curiosity to establish the nature of the disease prompted Dr George Thomson to carry out an autopsy on the body of a plague victim, whose skin was 'so beset with spots black and blew, more remarkable for multitude and magnitude than any I have yet seen'. Others noted the symptoms of the disease. Bing was confused by their variety: 'One week the general distempers are botches and boils; the next week as clear-skinned as may be... One week, full of spots and tokens; and perhaps the succeeding, none at all. Now taken with a vomiting and looseness, and within two or three days almost a general raging madness.' But, whatever the symptoms and speed of death, his conclusion was that 'Many are sick, and few escape'.

There was no shortage of advice on preventatives and medicines. The Privy Council directed the College of Physicians to issue, in English, advice and prescriptions, and its *Necessary Directions* included, among other suggestions, the lighting of fires and discharging of guns. The Council was keen on the idea of the fumigation of houses and recommended the practice to the justices. Its efficacy was demonstrated by James Angier, who burned a fumigant in houses in Newton Street, off High Holborn. This proved to be a success, for there were no further deaths in the houses that had been fumigated, although in one of them four people had died of the plague already and two more were infected. The Westminster justices were so impressed that they made a favourable report to the Privy Council, and a notice was issued listing five places where the 'Remedies & Medicaments with directions for the use of them may be had'. Angier himself was paid £86 'for fumes in the late sickness time', suggesting the use of his fumigants in more than just the few houses where they were first tested. And some householders fumigated their properties daily with fires and concoctions of herbs. In early September, the practice tried in earlier epidemics of burning fires in the streets, to prevent the air stagnating, was adopted, with one bonfire for every twelve houses. Rain fell after three days and doused the fires, and the operation was not renewed. Pepys was irritated by the rain, but not because of its effects on the fires: '...it being a most cursed rainy afternoon, having had none a great while before. And I, forced to go to the office on foot through all the rain, was almost wet to the skin, and spoiled my silk breeches, almost.'

The policy of public bonfires seems to have had little support and had not been tried earlier during this outbreak. Perhaps by the beginning of September the authorities were becoming desperate, as the statistics worsened. The number of recorded deaths from plague in the week ending 5 September was 6,988, with the figure for all deaths put at 8,252. Evelyn reported the number 'which the pestilence has mow'd downe in London this weeke' and suspected that there were 'possibly halfe as many more conceil'd'. The next week saw a fall, to 6,544 and 7,690, but the figures then rose again and the week ending 19 September saw 7,165 plague deaths and 8,297 in all. But this proved to be the peak, and the next week saw a drop to 5,533 and 6,460. There was then a steady fall in the numbers until the end of October.

Contemporaries anticipated such a pattern, partly from experience and partly because the numbers who had left or had died reduced the number of potential victims. A timely new edition of Graunt's *Natural and Political Observations* on the Bills of Mortality was issued. At its meeting on 20 June, the Royal Society agreed to suspend its weekly meetings until the epidemic came to an end; it also approved 'the reprinting of that book', with the additions seen by Sir William Petty. The principal addition was the appendix, with a consideration of London's population and the numbers of deaths in plague outbreaks in European cities, up to and including that in Amsterdam in 1664. The London returns were brought right up to date, with the figures from the Bills for 4 July. Pepys was given one of the 'new-printed and enlarged' copies on 25 July. Perusal of Graunt's tables would have shown that the peak for deaths in 1603 had been the week ending 1 September, and in 1625 it had come two weeks earlier. The numbers of deaths in those outbreaks had been considerably lower than in 1665, because of the city's smaller population. That was temporarily reduced in each plague year because of the retreat and death of so many citizens. A tax list for Westminster in 1665 suggests that twelve per cent of its inhabitants had gone away. Applying this proportion across the capital, and deducting the number of 'excess' deaths from May until the end of September, suggests that approximately 350,000 people remained.

The contemporary view that plague outbreaks declined because of the shrinking number of potential victims was partly based on an impression of depopulation, which came from changed patterns of behaviour by many of those who did not go away. With the court and fashionable society gone, there was less reason for stylish young gentlemen to disport themselves, and fewer customers for the prostitutes, as Thomas Vincent remarked, 'few ruffling gallants walk the streets; few spotted ladies to be seen at windows: a great forsaking there was of the adjacent places where the plague did first rage'. Others who did not need to go out and about were fastidious in taking care to limit their contacts and hardly stirred from their houses. Edward Wood's advice to his business partner, John Pack, was to 'Locke upp the Dores, &... goe abroad as litle as may be'. And so it seemed that the capital was almost deserted.

The effects of the epidemic on London's economy had become evident early on. In mid-June, as the number of plague deaths began to rise, John Moore, a merchant who imported and exported on a large scale, wrote that 'if the sicknesse increases we shall have nothing to doe for it will put a stopp to all businesse'. This was an accurate prediction, based on the memory of earlier epidemics. Six weeks later, the bishop of London's appeal for assistance described how there were 'many thousands of poore Artisans being ready to starve for Lacke of Meanes to be imployed in their Callings All Trading being become dangerous and layd aside by reason of the spreading of the Contagion'. The Dutch ambassador told the States General that many of his countrymen were asking for certificates so that they could leave, 'there being no trade left', nor company to converse with, at court or the Exchange. By the middle of August, Richard Fuller, a wine merchant in Mark Lane, found that he could not sell any goods or collect debts; only one merchant in 100 was left in the city, and the streets were so quiet that every day seemed like a Sunday.

In the middle of August, Pepys commented 'how sad a sight it is to see the streets empty of people, and very few upon the [Ex]Change'. Two months later, when the number of deaths was declining, he was again struck by the air of desertion as he walked through the City: 'But Lord, how empty the streets are, and melancholy... so many sad stories overheard as I walk, everybody talking of this dead, and that man sick, and so many in this place, and so many in that.' Vincent later recalled the 'dismal solitude in London's streets'; the shops were shut and the 'people rare and very few that walk about, insomuch that the grass begins to spring up in some places'. The rattling of coaches, the sound of horses and the enticing cries of street vendors had fallen silent.

Yet much normal business had to be carried on as before, albeit in a quieter and perhaps even furtive manner. Those who remained needed supplies and had to go out to obtain them. They could avoid others, walk in the centre of the streets, not talk to those they passed, enter a shop only when it contained no other customer and not accept money unless it had been soaked in vinegar. Shops were closed, for quarantine, or as their owners died or moved away, which perhaps would require longer journeys for customers than before. Pepys estimated that two-thirds of shops in his district were closed, and in October John Evelyn found those in the City 'universaly shut up'.

Servants should have been more vulnerable in these conditions than those householders with domestic help, who could send their maids, menservants or apprentices to run errands, rather than go out themselves. But this is not borne out by figures for the first victims to die of plague in households in a sample of eleven parishes. They show that fifteen per cent of them were servants, a lower proportion than in both 1603, when it had been twenty-seven per cent, and 1625, when the figure was eighteen per cent. The figures indicate a steady fall over the three major epidemics of the century and also show that the largest category of first victims in 1665 was children, who accounted for forty-one per cent of first deaths. Clarendon believed that the 'greatest number of those who died consisted of women and children'.

During the seventeenth century, the balance between the sexes coming to London was changing, with a rising demand for domestic servants, many of whom were female, and a relative decline in the number of male apprentices. The increase in female deaths is attested by returns from parishes in both the City and the outer areas, and may partly be accounted for by the vulnerability of domestic servants and those women housekeepers left alone in charge of houses when the families went away, and those who were pregnant. Infants, too, were put at risk from lack of proper care, as family routines were disrupted in households where plague was identified, as well as from the disease itself, and the number of deaths of children increased, indicated by the registers and the high proportion of first victims who fell into that category.

As well as those who necessarily maintained their usual routines, adapting them to minimise the danger, others bravely gave what help they could to the sick and bereaved, and the crisis did throw up cases of selfless devotion to duty. John Green, constable of High Holborn, was 'very vigilant and diligent in the performance of his office', making returns to the justices at least twice a week listing the visited houses, the numbers within them, how they were provided for and the cost of maintaining them, and he dipped into his own pocket to the extent that when he died the parish owed him £55. Among the conscientious clergymen was Simon Patrick, who thought that he had been fortunate to survive, considering 'how many dangers I had been in by people coming to speak to me out of infected houses, and by my going to those houses to give them money'. He visited the sick, distributing alms, and officiated at burials; he had to attend the interment of six victims during one night in mid-October.

Daniel Fervaques, a member of the French community, also took risks visiting houses so that the life of the community would continue to function. He was comfortably off and of some standing in London, as a Common Councilman and an Upper Bailiff of the Weavers' Company, yet not only did he stay in the city, but when the elder of the Blackfriars district died, Fervaques took the responsibility for distributing the tokens for the monthly communion. The wealthy Dutch merchant Willem de Visscher lived in the parish of St Mary at Hill, and, according to John Aubrey, 'stayed in London during the whole time of the Plague, and had not all that time one sick in his family. He was a temperate man, and had his house very cleanly kept.' The implication was that cleanliness contributed to freedom from the plague, but other members of the Dutch community did not escape. One of the ministers, Cesar Calandrini, reported on 21 September that a maid of his had caught the plague. He fell ill on the following day

and died on 26 September, and his fellow minister refused to
return from Barnes, where he was convalescing and claimed
to be suffering from a fever. He did not attempt to disguise
his fears, which had been increased by the fact that Calandrini
had died after moving into his house, supposedly of a fever not
plague, but 'It is sufficiently known that in times of plague, all
fevers are, to say the least, subject to suspicion.' Joas Evenson,
a wealthy merchant and deacon, had moved to Oxford and
he, too, declined to return, citing the deaths of two servants
during October and the misfortune of his maidservant who
was 'attacked by many ulcers' early in November, although
she recovered.

Senior parishioners, leading tradesmen and the incumbent
of the parish, took responsibility for listing the goods of a
deceased person, as part of the process of administering their
estate, if it was worth more than 50s. This was done to protect
the executors or administrators against excessive or false claims
upon the estate and safeguard the beneficiaries from fraud.
Many valuers went from room to room, often itemising the
deceased's belongings individually. There was an understandable reluctance to carry out this procedure in the house of
someone who had died of plague. After William Bull had died
in St Giles, Cripplegate, in September, the appraisers would
not compile a detailed probate inventory, but submitted to
the probate court a document which stated that he had died
possessed of 'goods and chattels to the value of aboute Thirty
pound but by reason the dec[ease]d dyed of the sickness the
same cannot as yet be vallued'.

Because of the scale of the mortality, not only routine procedures such as this but also the plague regulations were neglected,
even though many senior figures had not shirked their responsibilities and had remained behind. The presence of the Lord
Mayor, Sir John Lawrence, and some of the aldermen at the
Fast Day service mentioned by Bing shows that they were still

in London and not afraid to go into public places and assemble
in a congregation. Nevertheless, Lawrence was said by the
Venetian ambassador to have been cautious when transacting
business, having had a glass case made, from within which
he received visitors. The Archbishop of Canterbury, Gilbert
Sheldon, the bishop of London, Humphrey Henchman, the
Duke of Albermarle and the Earl of Craven also remained in
the capital, as did some of the parish clergy.

The Privy Council required nine named justices in
Westminster and the out-parishes to remain at their houses,
'to the end that the People may be the better governed, & such
Orders observed in this sad season as are necessary'. Among
their duties, they were to keep a note of those surgeons, physicians, apothecaries and others who were 'most eminent in
exposing themselves either by entring into infected Houses
for the better assisting infected Persons with proper Remedies
for preventing or curing the said sicknes, or doing any other
notable Service toward that end'. Their names were to be sent
to the king on his return to Whitehall after the epidemic, with
the promise of a reward over and above the sum that they
would have received, which 'in regard of the generall Calamity
is not like to be proportionable to their merit'. Evidently, a
financial carrot was felt to be necessary to enhance their sense
of duty.

Albermarle and Craven supervised the implementation of
the Privy Council's policies. Their task became increasingly
difficult, due to the sheer numbers infected and dying, and
the deaths of some of the parish officers who had to enforce
the plague orders and maintain the tally of the numbers of
deaths. Clarendon thought that the records must have been
deficient because 'The frequent deaths of the clerks and sextons of parishes hindered the exact account every week'. Both
of the churchwardens at St Bride's and three churchwardens
at St Giles, Cripplegate, died of the disease, and Simon Ford

found the burial of a sexton in a grave which he had dug a poignant one: 'The sexton oft the grave himself did fill, He'd digged for others'.

Craven's experience confirmed his belief that an epidemic could be checked in the early stages by the removal of infected cases to pesthouses, not by incarcerating them in their homes. Neither procedure could be effective when the outbreak developed. Indeed, the system of household isolation seems to have all but disintegrated as the number of sick rose. As early as 10 August, the justices were ordered to restrain those who refused to remain shut up, although someone in their family was infected, and on the following day John Allin wrote that he was fearful because of 'some piece of indiscretion used in not shutting up'. St Giles, Cripplegate, was so badly hit by the epidemic that household quarantine could not be maintained, as the parish lacked the means to provide essentials for the victims and their contacts. The district was a peculiar jurisdiction of the Dean of St Paul's and so John Tillison, the Clerk of Works, wrote to Sancroft on 15 August to tell him that 'the miserable condition of St Giles' Cripplegate... is more to be pitied than any parish in or about London, where all have liberty least their sick and poor should be famished within doors'. At the end of the month, 567 were recorded as dying of the plague in the parish in just one week. The Church distributed alms and within a week Tillison was able to dispense £5, authorised by Sancroft. But a further £40 could not be released when Dr Peter Barwick, brother of the late Dean, was taken so ill that he was in no condition to discuss the matter, nor did Tillison wish to risk going to see him. He went instead to the City financier Sir Robert Viner to draw on money which a Mr Welsteed had deposited with him, but Viner would not pay without a note from the depositor, which could not be obtained because he had left and all that was known of his whereabouts was that he was 'some where towards Uxbridge'. Viner was very correct in his response, although he could have acknowledged the urgency of the situation and the disruption caused by the epidemic by showing some flexibility.

As in earlier epidemics, collection of rates was difficult and charitable donations became essential to provide for those who were quarantined in their houses. Simon Patrick was helped by the £50 received from just one donor. The Earl of Bedford gave £10 each to Patrick and the vestry at St Margaret's, Westminster, and another £10 for building the pesthouse. But such donations were so uncertain and erratic that at St Giles, Cripplegate and elsewhere they were insufficient to enable the parish officers to maintain household quarantine. The Middlesex justices acknowledged this in the following February, when they made an order against inmates, echoing the comments of the Privy Council thirty years earlier, with the remark that 'the wealthy are not able to relieve the poore in time of health, much lesse in time of sicknesse or infeccion, as hath appeared in the late visitacion of the plague'.

In the middle of September, Pepys noted that he spoke to as few people as possible, as there was 'now no observation of shutting up of houses infected'. This is supported by Vincent's observation that 'shutting up of visited-houses (there being so many) is at an end, and most of the well are mingled among the sick'. This may have varied between the small City parishes with relatively manageable numbers of plague cases, where the orders could be observed, and the large ones around the fringe of the City where the parish administrations were under enormous pressure because of the size of the parishes, the numbers of sick, the difficulty of raising funds and the deaths of the parish officers. But even in the City, the arrangements were breaking down. In mid-October, when Pepys walked from the Tower to Lombard Street, then to the Royal Exchange at the junction of Threadneedle Street and Cornhill, before returning to the Tower, he encountered, 'so many poor sick people in the streets, full of sores', who should have been isolated.

At about the same time, John Evelyn went around the City on business and whenever he got out of his coach he found himself 'invironed with multitudes of poore pestiferous creatures, begging almes'. Simon Patrick also noted that 'In many Places they do not shut them up', and he was critical of those who did not stay in their houses as required, exhibiting a strong social prejudice in his criticism of those who came out even when they did not need to do so: 'where they ought to be more civill. But wee must not expect that from ordinary People: it is a Thing proper to better bred Souls. If the Vulgar be not intollerably rude, we are beholden to them.' On the other hand, some citizens were exasperated by the inconsistent application of the orders and the failure to close the houses of the elite. In September, four men were bound over to appear at the next Sessions for 'attempting to shut up' the Lord Mayor's house in St Helen's, Bishopsgate, presumably because, as he had been in contact with suspected plague victims, his house should have been quarantined, as others were in similar circumstances.

Clearly, some of the City parishes, as well as the poorer and more crowded ones, were overwhelmed by the scale of the disaster and could not maintain the quarantine system, even though they were not as badly affected as those in other parts of London. The ninety-seven parishes within the walls had 4.6 times the normal number of deaths in 1665. By contrast, on the north side of the City, in St Giles, Cripplegate and St Leonard, Shoreditch, the figure was 7.2 times the norm, and in the parishes of St Botolph-without-Aldgate and St Botolph-without-Bishopsgate, the multiple was 6.8. The East End parishes suffered almost as badly, with a crisis mortality ratio of 6.5, as did Southwark, where the comparable figure was 6.4. To the west of the City, the increase in deaths was

rather less: in Holborn and St Giles-in-the-Fields it was 5.7
and Westminster experienced a level of mortality that was 4.7
times the normal figure.

The size of the average household displays the differences
in wealth of these areas. This can be measured by the number
of hearths per household in the returns for the hearth tax,
which was introduced in 1662 and so provides evidence not
available for the earlier epidemics. For St Giles, Cripplegate,
St Leonard, Shoreditch, St Botolph-without-Aldgate and St
Botolph-without-Bishopsgate, the figure was 2.75 hearths; for
Stepney and Whitechapel it was 2.7; and for Southwark and
Bermondsey, 2.8. In the intramural parishes for which data
survive, the figure was significantly higher, at 4.7; to the west
of the City, in St Giles-in-the-Fields and St Andrew, Holborn,
it was higher again, at 5.1 hearths. The wealthiest area was St
Paul's Covent Garden, which had 7.7 hearths per household
and suffered only 3.2 times the average number of burials.
The contrast between wealthy and poor areas is also shown by
the figures for the average number of deaths per household.
In forty-two of the seventy-five parishes within the walls for
which the data are available, there were fewer burials than the
number of households, and in a sample of six of them the
average was 0.7 burials per household. In St Botolph-without-
Aldgate, however, the average was 2.5, and in Southwark the
figure was 1.2 burials for each household.

The actual numbers of burials indicate the extent of the
problem of disposal of the dead. During the previous five
years, the annual average number of burials for the whole of
the area within the Bills of Mortality was 14,229; yet in 1665
the figure was almost seven times higher. From the parishes
within the walls, 15,207 bodies had to be buried, but in the
four parishes on its north side, St Botolph-without-Aldgate
and St Botolph-without-Bishopsgate, St Giles, Cripplegate
and St Leonard, Shoreditch, the number of corpses was 19,128

and in Whitechapel and Stepney the figure was 13,364. At St Giles-in-the-Fields, the average number of burials in 1664 was fifteen per week, but in the summer of 1665 a far higher number of corpses was buried each day – more than thirty at the beginning of July and fifty-three on 21 July. The parishes were obliged to bury the bodies of those diagnosed as dying of plague as quickly as possible, while observing the requirements stipulated in the plague orders.

Early in August, John Allin commented on the practice of 'makeing great funeralls for such as dye of the distemper', and he was also alarmed because of 'a new burying place which they have made neere us'. At about the same time, Pepys became aware of burials being conducted during daylight hours, with 'the nights not sufficing to do it in', and also observed the numbers of people who were going to them, observing the normal social conventions in defiance of the orders. This was just what the plague policies were designed to avoid, and on 12 September, Clarendon, who was with the court at Oxford, sent a sharp response to Sheldon: 'that liberty you mention of visitinge each other, and goinge to publique buryalls must infecte the whole kingdome, and ought to be restrayned by the Magistrates, by all force & rigour. I have once more writt to my Ld Mayor, for whose remisnesse I am most sorry, the man beinge of excellent partes for government, and always reputed to be of good partes.' His intentions were all very well, but were somewhat detached from reality, as Bing explained to Sancroft, in a letter written two days after Clarendon's exasperated outburst. During the early stages of the epidemic, burials had been conducted at night, but now 'both night and day will hardly be time enough to do it. For the last week, mortality did too apparently evidence that, that the dead was piled in heaps above ground for some hours together, before either time could be gained or place to bury them in.'

Ground close to the new pesthouse in Soho Fields was used for burials and during the worst of the outbreak the dead were buried in pits, there and elsewhere. According to Thomas Rugge, each 'great hole' was filled with twenty, thirty or forty bodies, but when the number of deaths declined the dead were again interred in single graves. The burial place which concerned Allin contained a pit that was open daily and could be seen from his window. The pressure on the sextons and other parish officers was such that at times they could not deal with the numbers, and Clarendon later referred to 'the vast number that was buried in the fields, of which no account was kept'. Yet in one small City parish, all of the corpses were buried on the day of death or the following one, even though in the second half of the year the number interred was eleven times higher than normal.

Perhaps because of the bravado they displayed at a time when most people were subdued by fear and the sheer horror of the disaster, those who went around the city during the nights collecting bodies for burial drew some fierce criticism. Like the tolling of the bells, their necessary but gruesome task drew attention to the scale of the disaster and disconcerted the citizens by making them aware of the fragility of their own lives. John Tillison expressed this when he wrote to Sancroft: 'Death stares us continually in the face in every infected person that passeth by us; in every coffin which is daily and hourly carried along the street. The bells never cease to put us in mind of our mortality.' Rugge thought that those with the dead carts had themselves survived the plague and 'many of them was very idle base living men and very rude... a foul mouth crew'. Perhaps he found their lack of discernible gratitude for their deliverance offensive and, like Dekker, was disappointed that recovery from plague had not produced obvious evidence of a reformed life.

Others carrying out those tasks that involved direct contact with plague victims and the emergency relief efforts were castigated by contemporary writers. Nurses and searchers were alleged to steal from the sick and even to hasten the death of the plague sufferers, so that they could have the opportunity to rob their houses. Such hostility arose from the fact that they were poor men and women, often appointed from among those who received poor relief from the parish. In St Dunstan-in-the-West, one of the surveyors appointed by the vestry had been receiving payments in the previous winter, and the two searchers were both widows who received pensions from the parish. While, on the one hand, such people risked their lives carrying out the tasks required, on the other an epidemic gave them opportunities, access to houses and perhaps a purpose that would not otherwise have come their way, and at a time when supervision was loosened by the absence of those who normally kept tight control of parish matters.

Nurses were described as being negligent, the 'off-scouring of the City' who were 'dirty, ugly, and unwholesome Haggs', who frightened the patients rather than reassured them and were continually on the look-out to steal. To be ill and subject to the care of the parish was to risk being robbed by those designated as helpers. While Sarah Stapleton was lying sick of the plague in her house in East Smithfield, her goods were 'ransacked, pillaged and carryed away' by a woman and two men accomplices, who also prevented the constable and watchmen from entering. They, too, wanted to remove the goods, so that they could be sold and the money spent for Sarah's benefit, to 'keep her from being chargeable to the parish'. Even though the parish officers may have been under severe financial pressure in trying to provide for plague victims, the removal and sale of household effects from a house where someone was sick with the disease was contrary to the government's policy and the justices' instructions. Strict implementation of the orders was difficult in the pressured conditions of a full-blown epidemic, when the financial solutions were just not effective or were too slow in bringing in the required funds.

Among the plague victims was Dr Parker, the physician appointed by the City to take charge of the ward of Cripplegate Without and the parish of St Stephen, Coleman Street, and four women were later arraigned 'to aunswere the imbezilling the goods of Doctor Parker lately dead of the plague'. Disintegration of the social order was a concern during all major epidemics, which may explain the rather vehement reactions to such misconduct and petty crime. Yet some careful nursing was provided, because there were survivors, even in the pesthouses, where the numbers of sick and the crowded conditions might have made care difficult. Simon Patrick saw a group of about thirty people in the Strand early in September, carrying white sticks as they made their way from the pesthouse to the justices, who would provide them with certificates confirming their recovery. Early in 1666, St Thomas' Hospital donated £20 to Edward Rice, who had 'cured some officers and many patients of this disease, all the surgeons refusing to intermeddle therein'.

Criticism was directed not only at those poor people who held the posts connected to the outbreak and perhaps compensated themselves for the danger. Physicians and apothecaries also drew hostile comment, the physicians for leaving and the apothecaries, once again, for encroaching on the role of the physicians by treating the sick. They were also condemned for exploiting those who were ill, and increasing others' fears, by making unjustified claims for the efficacy of their medicines. The Privy Council was concerned that the citizens were 'being cheated by Counterfeit Remedies'. As in earlier outbreaks, a number of physicians remained behind – at least twenty-nine of them did so – and conscientiously treated the victims. But both the apothecaries and the so-called Chemical Physicians, such as George Thomson, their leading spokesman, were taking the opportunity provided by the crisis to attempt to improve their own professional positions and weaken the authority of the College. The apothecaries had already made progress in that respect and one of them, Nathaniel Upton, was well enough regarded to be appointed master of the City's pesthouse in Finsbury Fields.

The Chemical Physicians sought to demonstrate the validity of their theories and medical system, which were based on the writings of the early sixteenth-century Swiss physician Paracelsus and the Flemish chemist Jean Baptiste van Helmont. Thomson took the opportunity to castigate the members of the College and their continued observance of Galenist medicine, and explained that he could have left the city for the country 'as well as any Galenist', but would not do so and would risk his life because of 'the band of Charity towards my neighbour' and the disrepute which leaving brought upon the profession. A broadsheet issued as an advertisement by Thomson and colleagues, advocating their medicines, pointed out that the contagion was spreading 'notwithstanding the use of those common Galenical medicines, which have been recommended to the people by others'. But the deaths of some of the Chemical Physicians, such as Thomas O'Dowde, did not help their cause, demonstrating that their methods were not effective against plague, and Thomson's angry claims that the Galenist members of the College had left was only partly true. In any event, the College was too powerful, as well as strong in defence of its interests, to allow its position to be undermined by their actions during the outbreak.

The nonconformist clergy were also pursuing an anti-establishment agenda and hoped, by showing their willingness to stay to provide much-needed spiritual guidance, that the post-Restoration penal legislation would be reviewed and diluted. According to Gilbert Burnet, who was to be bishop of Salisbury under William III, 'several churches were

shut up, when people were in a more than ordinary disposition to profit by good sermons; whereupon some of the
Nonconformists went into the empty pulpits, and preached
with great freedom, reflecting on the vices of the Court
and the severities that they themselves had been made to
suffer'. Thomas Vincent approved of this process, justifying the
response of the unlicensed preachers on the grounds that the
churches were not being served and that this had produced a
critical reaction from those Londoners who remained, with
pamphlets appearing in the streets ironically drawing attention to those 'pulpits to be let'. At such a time, 'the law of God
and nature' took precedence over the laws of the state and
warranted preaching in the streets and in the pulpits of those
churches without clergy. He justified it, too, in terms of the
response of those Londoners who turned up in large numbers
to attend the services and hear the sermons, which were delivered by preachers animated by the dangerous circumstances
and so treating every sermon 'as if they were preaching their
last'. In mid-August, Bishop Henchman wrote that, 'Many
of those who never attended divine service are now present.'
Sometimes there were so many in the congregation that they
filled the aisles, and the preacher could get to the pulpit only
by climbing over the pews; the reaction was enthusiastic, with
the sermons producing 'such eager looks, such open ears, such
greedy attention, as if every word would be eaten which
dropped from the mouths of the ministers'.

Bing was not afraid to report this response to the negligence of the Anglican clergy to Sancroft, although expressing
it in hostile terms by complaining that in their sermons the
'monstrous spirits... will say that these Calamities are caused
by the Government in Church and State'. Tillison included in
one of his letters the remark that even those who were well
were frightened, on the one hand of being taken ill, and on
the other of 'the wicked inventions of hellish rebellious spirits

to put us in an uproar'. Undoubtedly, the nonconformists' reception by the congregations in the city reflected the earlier bonds between them, which caused misgivings among the ecclesiastical and political hierarchies. Henchman was concerned enough to order the Anglican clergy to return to their parishes, to fill the voids that were being exploited by the nonconformists, with the threat that they would lose their livings if they did not do so. And the laws against nonconformists were enforced, with those caught worshipping imprisoned, despite the danger from plague in the prisons.

Demonstration of the mutual loyalty between the nonconformist preachers and their congregations pointed to the need for stricter legislation to stem the criticism of the court and government from the pulpits, which smacked of the troubled years of Charles I's reign and the influence of the clergy on London's population, which had been critical of the court. This aspect of their role during the plague was the one which the government acted on, rather than rewarding their devotion to former congregations, and they produced further restrictive legislation, rather than an easing of the existing measures. The Five Mile Act was passed by the Oxford Parliament in 1665, designed to break this link, by banning all preachers and teachers who would not take the oaths and declaration required by the Act of Uniformity from coming within five miles of any corporate town or a parish where they had preached or taught.

Not all physicians, apothecaries and clergy who remained behind were acting out of a calculated self-interest, and some conscientiously stayed to do what they could to alleviate the suffering. Yet those professions were criticised for the response of some of their members, as was (once again) the household quarantine policy. The author of a pamphlet entitled *Golgotha, or a Looking-Glass for London* recognised the practice of shutting up houses to be the orthodox response, recommended by the

College of Physicians, but described this as the advice of four or five experts, which should be set against the experience of thousands of poor people. They were confined in small houses 'and with them an old woman, or some ignorant creature (a stranger to them as is usual) for their Nurse, and a sturdy fellow without with an Halberd (or some stricter Watch, as they have advised for others) to have to each of them no more than the Parish allows'. Many were taken by surprise and were confined without having been able to make practical provision by bringing in supplies, or prepare themselves for the ordeal of being separated from their normal social contacts. They were to remain in such conditions until forty days after the last death in the house. But the house was not truly sealed, for the doors were opened from time to time to admit the searchers and bearers, and food and drink were passed through the windows, and so the tainted air escaped. Worse still, it had become foul, and so more dangerous, because of the conditions created by keeping people together in 'such a nasty and infecting station'. Those who may have wished to help the quarantined were deterred from doing so because they thereby ran the risk of being confined themselves, and so, without help from those who were known to them, the sick and those shut in with them had to 'take any ignorant Nurse (or worse) in haste, to their great hazard'. And finally, the author appealed to the experience of earlier epidemics, when Londoners had been 'wearied out of this oppression'.

Another writer stressed the fact that one of the effects of household quarantine was to increase the danger. Those who discovered that they or someone in their family was infected absconded, rather than suffer the effects of being shut up. They then risked spreading the plague, by infecting those that they came into contact with as they went, 'scattering the infection along the streets... and shifting it from Lodging to Lodging' until they collapsed and died among strangers, putting them in jeopardy as well. In this way, the disease had been spread to the places around London, although if those who were at risk were allowed to take medicines and calmly consult with physicians and friends, they probably would be content to remain indoors and the objective of the policy would be achieved, without the disastrous consequences of the compulsory system.

Friends were kept apart from the infected and so prevented from helping them, producing ill-feeling, and the frenzy that sometimes afflicted the victims could cause them to attack their relatives who were incarcerated with them. A man in Fleet Lane who had 'a great Swelling, but not without hope of being almost ripe for breaking, did in a strong fit rise out of his bed, in spite of all that his Wife (who attended him) could do to the contrary, got his Knife, and therewith most miserably cut his Wife, and had killed her, had she not wrapped the sheet about her'. She was saved by her own swift reaction and that of a neighbour, who himself was shut up, yet heard her shouts and broke out of his own house and into hers to restrain her husband, who later died. Careful nursing and attention might have saved him, and others, had that been permitted. This incident may have been anecdotal, included to emphasise the lack of adequate support, but the author evidently believed it to be plausible, in the fearful atmosphere of the time.

Such objections were familiar from earlier epidemics, but did not lose effect from being repeated, and they convey the sense of horror, verging on terror, which came over those who were diagnosed as suffering from plague, or realised that a family member had fallen victim. The disease and its consequences, the prospect of confinement and heartless nursing by strangers: all generated dread. Rational decision-making must have been difficult at such a time, and the quarantine system was, indeed, designed to overcome hasty reactions by putting the isolation measures in place immediately. But this could not be done consistently in the face of opposition and, more than any other aspect of plague policy, household quarantine revealed the antagonism between authority and the community. The failure to enforce it effectively, given the scale of the outbreak and hostility, was blamed for the spread of the disease both during 1665 and 1666. After a summer of high mortality across much of England, in October 1666 Clarendon wrote that 'it is indeede a sadd season that wee are chased from one place to another to save our lyves. Wee have reason to complayne of the ill government of the citty of London, which, for want of shuttinge up infected houses, hath skattered the contagion over the kingdom.' Sir Thomas Peyton at Knowlton, in east Kent, was more specific, blaming the parish of St Giles-in-the-Fields: 'That one parish of St. Giles at London hath done us all this mischief'.

Clarendon expected the policy to be enforced, regardless of the fact that many Londoners were hostile to its implementation. It was restated in the orders sent to the City and Middlesex justices in February 1666, which repeated the requirement that those diagnosed as plague victims should be taken to the pesthouses, and the houses of those who could not be moved should be 'shutt up, & garded with a warder as formerly & a Red Crosse affixed upon the Doore'. When a house was opened, a white cross was to be attached to the door, with the date of the last death to have occurred there. This was to remain for a further forty days, during which time the house and contents were to be fumigated, first with brimstone and then 'other wholesome fumes'. Recognition of the inherent problems came with the direction that especial care should be given to 'such poore as shall be shutt up of the plague, in providing them mayntenance, Nurses & Warders'. But the regulations had to be reconsidered in the light of such a destructive epidemic. As in 1603 and 1625, Parliament turned its attention to plague in the immediate aftermath of the epidemic, and new plague orders were issued in May 1666, in which prominence was given to the removal of the sick to pesthouses as soon as the symptoms appeared. The emphasis on this aspect of the response to an outbreak of plague could have been designed to reduce resistance to the implementation of household quarantine, by going some way to meeting the complaints of those who pointed out that the effect of quarantining the healthy with the sick was to increase the number of deaths. Their swift removal would reduce that danger.

But were those fears justified? Was the practice of confining people together in a house for forty days or more as dangerous as the letter-writers and commentators suggested? This is difficult to assess. Certainly, entire households seem to have died from the disease in some cases, and they, quite understandably, attracted attention, yet it was far more common for there to have been only one or two victims. In a sample of six parishes in 1665, in almost two-thirds of affected households there was only one death, and in only five per cent were there more than three deaths. Mortality was higher in the alleys and courts, where roughly a third of Londoners lived, than in the main streets. But even so, in an alley off Fleet Street, in the twelve infected houses there was an average of only three deaths, and not all of the houses were closed.

If someone was infected outside the house and the other members of the household had not been exposed to infective fleas, then the disease would not be transmitted to them. And people may not be equally attractive to fleas. In April 1662, Pepys and a friend shared a bed in Portsmouth for the night, and the diarist noted 'that all the fleas came to him and not to me'. Mosquitoes with the parasite that carries malaria are drawn by the smell of some people, who produce an aroma in their sweat which the mosquitoes find attractive, while they are not enticed by others, whose smells are not appealing or who generate a masking odour. If the plague was in fact a contagious virus, not transmitted by fleas, it did not produce a very high mortality rate among close contacts. The proportion of the population who had contracted the disease and recovered cannot be estimated, but they may account for some of the survivors in the quarantined houses. Others may have carried an inherited immunity, although this should have increased the survival rate of children, inheriting from one, perhaps both, parents, yet the mortality level among children rose considerably during this epidemic, as in earlier ones.

Despite the survival of so many potential victims, across the whole of London for the period of just less than a year, from 27 December 1664 to 19 December 1665, the Bills recorded 97,306 deaths, 88,395 of them after the end of May and 68,956 attributed to plague. Almost certainly, the number of plague deaths was under-recorded. This had occurred in previous epidemics, through deliberate falsification of the cause of death, which was widely thought to have been practised again during the Great Plague. The nature of the Bills, as a record of plague deaths in particular, and the process by which they were compiled, invited such deceit, as part of the general unwilling-ness to observe the regulations for quarantining households. Deaths from other causes showed considerable increases, with a twentyfold rise in the number attributed to spotted fever during the summer months. The pattern of non-plague deaths was similar to that of deaths from plague, rising during the summer months and peaking in late August and early September. Some of those deaths must have been caused by plague and the attributions to other diseases, especially fever and spotted fever, were deliberately false in those cases. In addi-tion, nonconformists, members of the Huguenot and Dutch congregations, and Jews, who had been allowed to return to England in 1656, were outside the parochial system and so their deaths were not registered, although the Quakers recorded

1,177 deaths. The Jewish community numbered fewer than 300 at the Restoration and may have increased by 1665, before being reduced by the plague. Attendance at the synagogue in Creechurch Lane in the spring of 1666 was said to have been 'much diminished'.

The true figure for plague deaths probably was in excess of 70,000 and perhaps as many as 75,000, with more than 100,000 deaths from all causes by 19 December, roughly twenty per cent of the total population and six times the average for the past ten years. And the epidemic continued through the winter and into 1666, with 1,800 plague burials during that year in London. Many communities in southern and eastern England, as far north as the River Tyne, suffered from the epidemic in the mid-1660s, experiencing higher mortality in 1666 than in 1665. Colchester, Norwich, Winchester and Southampton suffered especially high mortality, while the reaction to the disease by the inhabitants of the Derbyshire village of Eyam, who agreed to remain within the parish rather than flee and risk spreading the disease, has become celebrated.

The outbreaks elsewhere during the middle years of the decade added to London's economic problems, with interruptions in the supply of goods and raw materials. Overseas trade was suspended, with incoming ships detained at the quarantine station, and outgoing cargoes held up at their destination for the same process, if they were received at all. Trade with the United Provinces was at a standstill because of the war and Dutch privateers preyed on British shipping, capturing as many as 500 vessels and intercepting ships bound for or leaving British ports, whether sailing under the British flag or not. English vessels sailing eastwards through the Danish Sound into the Baltic averaged ninety-one per year in 1661–64, but the number then fell to twenty-three in 1665, none in 1666 and five in 1667, before rising again and averaging ninety-three in 1668–71.

The decline in trade reduced the sums received by the customs officers and, as in earlier epidemics, the collection of taxes, both local and national, was extremely difficult. London's contribution to the exchequer was so great that this was bound to have an effect on the funding of the war against the Dutch, who were joined by the French in January 1666. The plight of the wounded sailors and prisoners became desperate because of the shortage of funds for provisions and care, although the fleet could be equipped and was able to operate, and the plague did not spread to the crews. As in 'the great plague' of 1625, a major epidemic in the capital had coincided with a naval campaign. But mortality in the outbreak in 1665 far exceeded that forty years earlier and so it now took the title of the Great Plague.

Despite the scale of the outbreak in 1665, during the late seventeenth century the epidemic forty years earlier was still remembered when a recurrence of plague was feared. In 1680, John Aubrey noted with concern that 'Mr Fabian Philips sayes the winter 1625 before the Plague was such a mild winter as this'. Aubrey also noted that William Camden included in his *Britannia* (1586) 'a remarkable Astrologicall observation, that when Saturn is in Capricornus a great Plague is certainly in London. He had observed it all his time, and setts downe the like made by others before his time. Saturn was so posited in the great plague 1625, and also in the last great plague 1665.'

But awareness of the epidemic in 1625 and the earlier outbreaks gradually receded, while the epidemic in 1665 continued to attract much attention, because of its scale, the fact that it proved to be the last outbreak in London, and, not least, through two of Daniel Defoe's works which dealt with it, *Due Preparations for the Plague* and the far more popular and influential *A Journal of the Plague Year*. Both books appeared in 1722, among a flurry of publications issued in response to the outbreak of plague in Provence, which began in 1720 and claimed the lives of roughly a half of the inhabitants of Marseille, producing high levels of mortality in Toulon, Arles, Aix-en-Provence and other towns in the region. Their authors naturally looked back to the epidemic in 1665, which Defoe described as 'the most violent infection that ever yet happened in this nation'. Indeed, the Great Plague came to be regarded as the only significant visitation of plague in London since the Black Death, rather than as the last and most destructive of a number of major outbreaks.

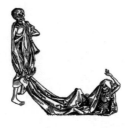

6

Metropolis and Plague

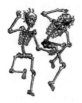

A possible outcome of the effects of plague in Tudor and Stuart London could have been a city reeling under the periodic shocks of at least one epidemic in every generation, each killing about a fifth of the population; trade coming to a virtual standstill while the outbreak lasted and limping along in other years when the plague was raging elsewhere; industry blighted by breaks in the supply of raw materials and disruption to markets, exacerbated by the loss of both skilled and unskilled labour. And underlying this, there could have been seething social resentment and discontent, aggravated by the flight of many of the wealthy and responsible citizens, and manifested by blatant defiance of the regulations imposed during plague outbreaks. Added to the problems caused by the pestilence were the disruption and economic harm that resulted from the Civil Wars in the 1640s, the three Dutch Wars between 1652 and 1674, and the Great Fire in 1666, the most destructive accidental fire in the history of western Europe, with more than 13,000 houses destroyed.

Surely this death, disruption and destruction could have produced an economic downturn, with a falling population: the birth rate insufficient to replace the losses, and migrants reluctant to come to such a dangerous place, with the Bills of Mortality providing not only warnings of the early stages of an epidemic, so that countermeasures could be put in place, as was intended, but, more negatively, the evidence to excite the fears of those who were considering moving to the metropolis. The scarcity of labour that would ensue would create wage infla-tion, which, added to the rising prices caused by the shortage of raw materials, must damage the city's competitiveness, lead to the departure of merchants to rival cities and so generate a spiral of decline.

But this did not happen; the seemingly great disasters did not produce such detrimental consequences, certainly in the long term, or even in the short term. London experi-enced particularly rapid expansion between about 1560 and 1640 – that is, during the period when plague was taking a heavy toll – and continued to grow throughout the rest of the seventeenth century, despite the Great Plague. By 1700, roughly one in ten English people lived in the capital and its population may have been as high as 575,000, compared to 50,000 in 1500. John Graunt's conclusion that London's population recovered to its previous level by the second year after the major epidemics in 1603 and 1625 also held good after the much higher mortality in 1665. Despite the numbers killed and the destruction of housing by the conflagration in the following year, the population probably was back to its pre-plague level by 1667 and was larger in the late 1660s than it had been in the early years of the decade.

After each disaster, the court and the merchants returned and business revived; cloth from the producing areas could be moved to London once restrictions were eased, and non-perishable goods that had been held back were also shipped in and out of the capital. Even so, that process would not in itself have generated a full economic recovery if the disease had been so widely feared that the capital was shunned. But the anxieties of some contemporaries, who were shocked by its horrible effects on individual victims, as well as being aware of the scale of its impact, could not have been widely shared once the number of deaths declined and the danger receded. After all, roughly eighty per cent of the citizens survived even the most destructive outbreaks, and the majority of them had remained in London. Others soon returned. Observers were not aware of a continuing stream of departures as an outbreak subsided; instead they noted the early, sometimes fatally premature, return of those who had left and of others who moved in during the epidemic, drawn partly by the chance of occupying empty houses and carrying out functions vacated by those who had fled or died. Their behaviour was deplored, though they surely helped to maintain a higher level of activity than if the movement had been only outwards, away from London, and a speedy recovery as an epidemic declined. Early in September 1625, the city at one o'clock in the afternoon was no busier than it would have been at three o'clock on a summer morning in normal times, 'no more people stirring, no more shops open', yet only six weeks later an increase in plague deaths was feared, 'by reason of the wonderful number of people in the city... the streets full of people, and the highways of passengers – horse and foot'.

Not all parts of the capital or sections of society suffered equally. Although the City was affected in the sixteenth-century epidemics, during those in the seventeenth century it gradually became relatively less dangerous, with a far lower incidence of plague deaths there than in the outer areas. In any case, plague developed the reputation of being a disease of the poor, children and the elderly, living in back alleys and courts. From experience or collective memory, those who were considering moving to London would have been able to assess the risks and, if they had access to the Bills, to interpret them in a rational way. They showed that a year of high mortality from plague was never followed in the next year by equal mortality from the disease and that, commonly, the numbers of plague deaths in that year was relatively low. Furthermore, after a major outbreak there was then an interval of several years before another one struck with equal harshness. Surviving an epidemic gave a certain security for the immediate future. And fears of infection could also be qualified by the kind of employment that incomers expected to take.

However fearful people were, the death-toll from plague created opportunities. The sheer economic pull of London's burgeoning economy drew in those looking for employment, especially the young from south and east England. In normal non-plague years, the capital needed immigrants to sustain its size, and it got them. After a plague epidemic it needed far more, and yet it got them, too, despite the numbers involved and the recent disaster. Gregory King calculated that late-seventeenth-century London required an annual inflow of 2,000 immigrants just to maintain its population and 5,000 to sustain its current growth rate. After an epidemic, the need was measured in tens of thousands, but was achievable because London had no rival that could provide opportunity and employment on a similar scale for those seeking to advance their prospects or unable to obtain work locally. By the end of the seventeenth century, the combined populations of Norwich and Bristol were only seven per cent of that of London. And so the long-term demographic consequences of plague are to be found not only in

London, but also across south-east England, which lost many of its young people to the growing metropolis, and further afield, with migrants drawn from much of the British Isles.

The epidemics also set in train a demographic process that helped to stimulate the recovery of the city's population, because many Londoners whose spouse had died would remarry and start a new family, or parents of childbearing age who had lost children would have more. The peak in the number of burials during an epidemic was followed by a peak in marriages and then a rise in the number of births, above the pre-plague level. And so the generation that had suffered losses to plague may have produced more children than if it had not endured that experience.

Not only could the risks from plague be realistically assessed in the aftermath of an epidemic year, but so could concerns regarding the mood of the citizens, for migrants to London did not arrive in a city seething with discontent, whatever the reactions during the crisis itself. The effects of the major eruptions of plague might have had the potential to create such deep divisions in society that they failed to heal afterwards, producing a turbulent and potentially dangerous community, but this did not develop. In some ways, the effect of an outbreak of plague was to lay bare the structure of society, with its inherent inequalities, divisions and resentments exposed – the wealthy suffering much lower levels of mortality than the poor, because they had no compunction in leaving, and the departure of some of the clergy and other senior groups in society drawing rancour and contempt from those who had to stay. Yet such tensions did not become serious or damaging enough to harm the city's recovery. Indeed, its revival and return to normal seem to have been expected, and the epidemics did not produce a pessimistic reaction among its citizens, any more than it did among would-be immigrants.

Niccolò Molin, the Venetian ambassador, reached London in mid-December 1603, just as the epidemic was subsiding, and found that 'No one ever mentions the plague, no more than if it had never been. The City is so full of people that it is hard to believe that about sixty thousand deaths have taken place.' His figure for the number of deaths was exaggerated, but the proportion of the population that died in that outbreak was broadly similar to that in 1665, when Thomas Sprat, a Fellow of the Royal Society, was equally surprised at the citizens' positive response:

> Upon our return after the abating of the Plague, what else could we expect, but to see the streets unfrequented, the River forsaken, the fields deform'd with the Graves of the Dead, and the Terrors of Death still abiding on the faces of the living? But instead of such dismal sights, there appear'd almost the same throngs in all publick places, the same noise of business, the same freedom of convers, and with the return of the King, the same cheerfulness returning on the minds of the people as before.

This suggests that Pepys' memory of that awful time was not unusual, for when he summarised the year, he recalled that 'I have never lived so merrily... as I have done this plague-time'. He made that entry at the end of December, when he was pleased to note that 'the town fills apace, and shops begin to be open again'. Nor, in the longer term, was he able to discern any major economic damage from the plague, the Great Fire, or the Second Dutch War, for when he discussed the matter with Sir George Carteret in September 1667, they agreed that they could not recall having heard of any substantial citizen who had gone bankrupt. And after the mid-1660s the threat of plague disappeared, for the Great Plague proved to be the last epidemic in London, with the final deaths from the disease recorded at Rotherhithe in 1679.

London's role as national capital, and the increasing breadth of its economy, undoubtedly helped it to ride out a crisis. Smaller cities, with an over-reliance on one trade or function that was in decline, were more likely to suffer long-term effects from the dislocation that an epidemic brought in its train, although those which were prosperous before the plague struck were less vulnerable. Norwich's thriving cloth industry drove its economy and the city continued to grow throughout the sixteenth and early seventeenth centuries, despite periodic plague epidemics, and Colchester recovered fully from the terrible outbreak there in 1665–66.

Within the European context, London's experience resembles that of Amsterdam, which boomed after Antwerp's capture by the Spanish in 1585 caused a burst of emigration and loss of international trade. Amsterdam benefited, both from receiving many of the migrants and from a transfer of trade, and its population grew from 27,000 in 1560 to 120,000 by the mid-1630s and 200,000 by 1672, despite 94,500 plague deaths between 1624 and 1664. It owed its prosperity to the expanding economy of the United Provinces and its role as the leading port in a country that rapidly developed a dominant role in world trade in the late sixteenth and early seventeenth centuries. As in London, the last epidemic, in 1663–64, was the most destructive, but it did not check the city's growth.

By contrast, the Mediterranean cities suffered a net loss of population in the early seventeenth century, and the only ports on its coasts that grew during the century were Livorno and Malaga. Many of them suffered from the plague epidemics in the 1630s and 1650s. Venice's population did recover to its former level after the epidemic of 1630–31, thanks largely to immigration, but the process took almost twenty years. This was impressive, yet was a slower revival than after the equally severe outbreak in 1575–76, at a time when its economy was more flourishing than it was to be fifty years later, and distinctly sluggish compared with London and Amsterdam.

The plague could expose and perhaps accelerate existing trends, but it did not initiate them. London's economic and political dominance was not threatened by the successive outbreaks; Antwerp was the victim of political and military policies, not plague; the trade of Venice and Genoa was in relative decline before those cities were hit by the terrible outbreaks of the seventeenth century; and Amsterdam grew enormously, despite periodic epidemics. The collective reaction of the citizenry and potential immigrants from the countryside to such disasters contributed to the speed of recovery, as did the political response. But even when there was a positive reaction, such as that at Genoa after horrific losses in the epidemic in 1656, this could not overcome the difficulties of inherent structural weaknesses in a city's economy, especially when so many had died. There, and in other Mediterranean cities during the mid-seventeenth century, the proportion of the population that was lost during plague outbreaks was far higher than in any epidemic in London after 1500.

And so London emerged as a prosperous city from the long period of more than 300 years that was punctuated by plague epidemics. But why did they come to an end, especially so abruptly? Not because of the Great Fire in 1666, which destroyed only a part of the City, and not those districts around it and the suburbs that had been most badly affected in the previous year. The enforced rebuilding of the burnt area in bricks and tiles need not have had an effect, for few buildings are resistant to rats, and softwoods came into increasing use in building, in place of hardwoods. Nor did they end because of a change in the predominant species of rat, for both *rattus rattus* and the brown rat, which supplanted it in the British Isles during the eighteenth century, can carry infective fleas. Growing resistance to the disease among Londoners may have been a factor, but if the depredations of the sixteenth and seventeenth centuries had carried off that section of the population which had no resistance to plague, and left those who had such a resistance, the pattern would have been one of slowly diminishing peaks, as the proportion of the citizens with inherited immunity increased, rather than an abrupt end after the worst outbreak of all. Improved cleanliness of people, houses and public places would have had a similar, gradual effect.

So long as no cases of the disease were recorded in London, the difficult, contentious and socially divisive policy of household quarantine did not have to be put to the test. And as the danger of plague receded, it could even be treated facetiously. In *The Plain Dealer* (1676), William Wycherley's character Manly, troubled by an unwanted and persistent visitor, comments that 'I'd sooner be visited by the plague, for that only would keep a man from visits and his doors shut.' Nor was it necessary to reintroduce the inconsistent strategy of banning the congregation of people at fairs, plays, sports and funerals, while encouraging them to gather at church services. Other proposals for tackling plague and related areas of public health, such as the creation of health boards, had been defeated not by the opposition or scepticism of the citizens but by the reluctance of the City's government to adopt them, and the divided structure of London's administration.

In any case, policy had not been smoothly translated into practice. London's experience during the outbreaks of plague shows that for any policy to be effective, stringent application of the orders and dire penalties for defaulters were not enough without adequate finance and the compliance of the population, and neither were achieved. Many Londoners were reluctant to observe the plague orders, even during the major epidemics, either through fatalism or a conviction, based upon experience, that plague was not contagious. Some courageous people were in contact with those suffering from the disease and survived, including Henry Morse; others, such as John Boston, laboured among its victims for a number of weeks, but eventually succumbed. Going away ensured safety; remaining and living with the sick, or nursing them, may or may not have been fatal. Contemporaries generally did not react as though they had complete faith in the measures imposed by the government, City, justices and parishes. These may have been successful in containing outbreaks on a number of occasions, perhaps limiting the severity of those in 1636 and during the 1640s, but they failed to check the major epidemics in 1603, 1625 and 1665, which were as severe as those before the introduction of a systematic policy. Some Londoners preferred the interpretation which attributed plague epidemics to divine retribution upon a sinful and unrepentant city. No official policies could assuage that; remorse and reformation were needed.

The controls imposed on shipping probably explain the end of the outbreaks in England. They had saved London from the epidemics on the near continent in the 1650s, and throughout 1663 and 1664; the Scottish Privy Council imposed a quarantine on all vessels from England in 1665, and Scotland escaped that epidemic. The Great Plague in London may have originated from a vessel which slipped through the cordon, or because the controls were imposed after the bacillus had reached the city, the epidemic erupting only when the conditions became favourable. This was a potential flaw in shipping quarantine, that the authorities could put it in place only when the danger was apparent, for to act too soon would have risked arousing the antagonism of the merchants, and so evasion of the naval blockade. Defoe was aware that 'The Damage of obliging Ships to Quarantine, is... very considerable to the Merchants', and he feared that 'if one Villain can pass the Barriers set, – if one Man can escape out of these Ships, with a Parcel of any sort of Goods, dangerous to Health, he may lodge the Plague among us'.

But when Amsterdam and the other ports in northern Europe that traded with London succeeded in preventing outbreaks, the risk was much diminished, as voyages from more distant ports were fewer and so easier to control, acting upon intelligence from the places of origin of the potential danger of plague. Such controls could provide an effective barrier against the disease, as they were adopted more widely and extended by restrictions imposed along land frontiers, especially those of the Austrian empire. The pattern of the ending of plague outbreaks does support that hypothesis, with a gradual withdrawal south-eastwards within Europe. In the 1780s, Edward Gibbon, in his magisterial *The Decline and Fall of the Roman Empire*, referred to 'those salutary precautions to which Europe is indebted for her safety' from plague.

The reduction of plague epidemics in Europe was a more prolonged process than London's experience would suggest, and outbreaks elsewhere continued to have an effect on its economy, through their disruption of trade, and the consciousness of its citizens. Because of its impact, the numbers of its victims, the foulness of the disease, and the literature which it generated, plague cast a very long shadow. Towards the end of the eighteenth century, the image of plague depicted by William Blake, in his *Europe a Prophecy*, shows a sombre-looking bellringer in black walking past a man dragging away the corpse of a woman, while another woman laments; etched on the door in the background are the words 'Lord have mercy on us'. Although plague has not been a killer in London for more than 300 years, its reputation is such that it still makes headlines and still has the capacity to frighten us.

Bibliography

Sources

PRINTED SOURCES

Acts of the Privy Council
Bailey, Charles, *Transcripts from the Municipal Archives of Winchester* (1856)
Bédoyère, Guy de la, *Particular Friends: The Correspondence of Samuel Pepys and John Evelyn* (Boydell, 1997)
Beer, E.S. de, ed., *The Diary of John Evelyn* (Oxford University Press, 1959)
Calendars of State Papers, Domestic
Calendars of State Papers, Venetian
Chambers, E.K., and Greg, W.W, eds, *Dramatic Records of the City of London* (Malone Society Collections, vol.I (1907)
Cool, Jacob, *Den Staet van London in hare Groote Peste* (1962)
The Court and Times of Charles I, ed. R.F. Williams, 2 vols (1848)
Dick, Oliver Lawson, ed., *Aubrey's Brief Lives* (Penguin Books, 1972)
Ellis, Henry, *Original Letters Illustrative of English History*, 2nd series, vol.IV (1827)
Fookes, R.A., *Henslowe's Diary* (2nd edn, Cambridge University Press, 2002)
Freshfield, Edwin, ed., *The Vestry Minute Book of The Parish of St. Margaret Lothbury in the City of London 1571–1677* (1887)

Gough, John, *Chronicle of the Grey Friars of London* (Camden Soc., 1852)

Hall, A. Rupert, and Hall, Marie Boas, eds, *The Correspondence of Henry Oldenburg,* vol.II (University of Wisconsin Press, 1966)

Historical Manuscripts Commission, *Calendar of the Manuscripts of the Marquess of Salisbury* (HMSO, 1883–1976)

Historical Manuscripts Commission, *Calendar of the Manuscripts of the College of Physicians* (8th report, appendix, 1881)

Howarth, R.G., ed., *Letters and the Second Diary of Samuel Pepys* (Dent, 1933)

Inderwick, F.A., ed., *A Calendar of the Inner Temple Records,* I 1505-1603 (The Inner Temple, 1896)

Journals of the House of Commons

Journals of the House of Lords

Latham, Robert and Matthews, William, eds, *The Diary of Samuel Pepys,* Vol.6 (Bell, 1972)

The Letters and Papers of Henry VIII

Longstaffe, W.H.D., ed., *Memoirs of the Life of Mr. Ambrose Barnes* (Surtees Soc., L, 1867)

McMurray, William, ed., *The Records of Two City Parishes* (Hunter & Longhurst, 1925)

Middlesex County Records, vol.III, ed. J.C. Jeaffreson (Middlesex County Records Soc., 1888)

Mynors, R.A.B., and Thomson, D.F.S., *The Correspondence of Erasmus,* vol.II (University of Toronto Press, 1975)

Nevinson, Charles, *Later Writings of Bishop Hooper* (Parker Soc., 1852)

Nicholson, Watson, *The Historical Sources of Defoe's Journal of the Plague Year* (Stratford, 1919)

Nicholson, William, *The Remains of Edmund Grindal, D.D.* (Parker Soc., 1843)

Overall, W.H., *Analytical Index to the... Remembrancia... A.D. 1579 1664* (E.J. Francis, 1878)

Proceedings in Parliament 1625, ed. Maija Jansson and William B. Bidwell (Yale University Press, 1987)

Tudor Royal Proclamations (Yale University Press, 1964–9); *Stuart Royal Proclamations* (Oxford University Press, 1973–83), ed. P.L. Hughes and J.F. Larkin

Wilson, F.P., ed., *The Plague Pamphlets of Thomas Dekker* (Oxford University Press, 1925)

MANUSCRIPT SOURCES

Bodleian Library, MS.Add.c.303, the letters of the Earl of Clarendon

British Library, Thomas Rugge, '*Mercurius Politicus Redivius*', Add.MS 10,117

Lambeth Palace Library, Sheldon's Register
London Metropolitan Archives, Corporation of London Records
Common Council Journals; Aldermen's repertories
Middlesex Quarter Sessions records, WC/R, WJ/SP
Description of Clerkenwell, acc/1876/D1/A/1
Letters of Edward Wood, acc.262
St Saviour's Southwark *v.* Robert and Sarah White, P92/SAV/799-800 (1625)
The National Archives, Public Record Office, Privy Council Registers, PC2
Submission of Sir Theodore de Mayerne, SP16/533/17
A Short Proposall... for the Prevention of the Plague, SP29/122/123
Accounts of the Carthusian Priory, SC12/25/55
Wellcome Institute for the History of Medicine, Letter of John Moore, Western MS 7382/3

CONTEMPORARY WORKS

Anon., *A Treatise Concerning the Plague and the Pox* (1652)
Anon., *A Damnable Treason, By a Contagious Plaster of a Plague Sore... sent unto Mr. Pym* (1641)
[Ashmole, Elias, and Lilly, William], *The Lives of the Eminent Antiquaries Elias Ashmole, Esquire, and Mr. William Lilly, written by themselves* (1774)
Balmford, James, *A Short Dialogue concerning the Plagues Infection* (1603)
Bell, John, *London's Remembrancer: or, A true Accompt of every particular Weeks Christnings and Mortality In all the Years of Pestilence* (1665)
Boghurst, William, *Loimographia* (1894)
Bradwell, Steven, *A Watch-Man for the Pest* (1625)
Howes, John, *A Famyliar and Frendly Discourse...,* in Tawney, R.H., and Power, E., *Tudor Economic Documents*, vol.III (Longmans, 1925)
Cooke, John, *Unum Necessarium: Or, The Poore Mans Case* (1648)
Donne, John, *After Our Dispersion by the Sickness* (1625)
Dugdale, Gilbert, *The Time Triumphant* (1604) in *An English Garner*, ed. Edward Arber (Constable, 1903)
Evelyn, John, *Fumifugium* (1661) in *The Writings of John Evelyn*, ed. Guy de la Bédoyère (Boydell, 1995)
Graunt, John, *Natural and Political Observations... upon the Bills of Mortality* (1676) in *The Economic Writings of Sir William Petty* (Cambridge University Press, 1899)
Holland, Henry, *Spirituall Preservatives against the Pestilence* (1603)
I.D., *Salomon's Pest-House, Or Towre-Royall* (1630)
Jones, John, *A Dial for all Agues* (1566)
The Kings Maiesties Speech... to the Lords (1603)

Lodge, Thomas, *A Treatise of the Plague* (1603)

Mayerne, Theodore de and Cademan, Thomas, *The Distiller of London* (1652)

More, Thomas, *Utopia* (Dent, 1994)

Paynell, Thomas, *Moche profitable treatise against the pestilence* (1534)

Peter, Hugh, *Good Work for a Good Magistrate* (1651)

Petowe, Henry, *The Countrie Ague, Or, London her Welcome home to her retired Children* (1625)

Phayre, Thomas, *Treatise of the Pestilence* (1545)

Sherwood, Thomas, *The Charitable Pestmaster, Or, The Cure of the Plague* (1641)

Spencer, Benjamin, *Vox Civitatis, or Londons Complaint against her Children in the Countrey* (1625, reprint, University of Exeter, 1976)

Sprat, Thomas, *The History of the Royal Society of London* (1667)

Taylor, John, *The Fearfull Summer: Or, Londons Calamitie* (1625)

Vincent, Thomas, *God's Terrible Voice in the City* (1667, reprint Soli Deo Gloria, 1997)

Wheeler, John, *A Treatise of Commerce* (1601) in R.H. Tawney and E. Power, *Tudor Economic Documents*, vol.III (Longmans, 1925)

Books

Adams, Reginald H., *The Parish Clerks of London* (Phillimore, 1971)

Barroll, Leeds, *Politics, Plague, and Shakespeare's Theater: The Stuart Years* (Cornell University Press, 1991)

Beier, A.L. and Finlay, Roger, *London 1500–1700: The Making of the Metropolis* (Longman, 1986)

Bell, Walter, *The Great Plague in London in 1665* (John Lane, 1924; reprint, Bracken Books, 1994)

Benedictow, Ole, *The Black Death 1346–1353: The Complete History* (Boydell, 2004)

Bernard, G.W. and Gunn, S.J., *Authority and Consent in Tudor England* (Ashgate, 2002)

Braddick, Michael J., *State Formation in Early Modern England c.1500–1700* (Cambridge University Press, 2000)

Capp, Bernard, *When Gossips Meet: Women, Family, and Neighbourhood in Early Modern England* (Oxford University Press, 2003)

Caraman, Philip, *Henry Morse: priest of the plague* (Longmans, 1957)

Carlin, Martha, *Medieval Southwark* (Hambledon Press, 1996)

Chambers, E.K., *The Elizabethan Stage*, vol.IV (Oxford University Press, 1923)

Champion, J.A.I., ed., *Epidemic Disease in London* (Centre for Metropolitan History, 1993)

Champion, J.A.I., *London's Dreaded Visitation: The Social Geography of the Great Plague in 1665* (Historical Geography Research Series, No.31, 1995)

Cohn, Samuel K., *The Black Death transformed: disease and culture in early Renaissance Europe* (Arnold, 2001)

Cook, Judith, *Dr Simon Forman: A most notorious physician* (Chatto & Windus, 2001)

Creighton, Charles, *A History of Epidemics in Britain from A.D. 664 to the extinction of plague* (Cambridge University Press, 1891; Cass, 1965)

De Vries, Jan, *European Urbanization 1500–1800* (Harvard University Press, 1984)

Finlay, Roger, *Population and Metropolis: The Demography of London 1580–1650* (Cambridge University Press, 1981)

Forbes, Thomas Rogers, *Chronicle from Aldgate: Life and death in Shakespeare's London* (Yale University Press, 1971)

Griffiths, Paul and Jenner, Mark S.R., eds, *Londinopolis: Essays in the cultural and social history of early modern London* (Manchester University Press, 2000)

Gurr, Andrew, *Playgoing in Shakespeare's London* (2nd edn, Cambridge University Press, 1996)

Gwyn, Peter, *The King's Cardinal. The rise and fall of Thomas Wolsey* (Barrie & Kenkins, 1990)

Gwynn, Robin, *Huguenot Heritage: The history and contribution of the Huguenots in Britain* (2nd edn, Sussex Academic Press, 2001)

Healy, Margaret, *Fictions of Disease in Early Modern England: Bodies, Plagues and Politics* (Palgrave, 2001)

Inwood, Stephen, *A History of London* (Macmillan, 1998)

Local Population Studies, *The Plague Reconsidered: A new look at its origins and effects in 16th and 17th Century England* (Local Population Studies Supplement, 1977)

McNeill, William H., *Plagues and Peoples* (Doubleday, 1977)

Medvei, Victor Cornelius and Thornton, John L., eds, *The Royal Hospital of Saint Bartholomew 1123–1973* (Saint Bartholomew's Hospital, 1974)

Moote, A. Lloyd and Moote, Dorothy C., *The Great Plague: The Story of London's Most Deadly Year* (Johns Hopkins University Press, 2004)

Mullett, Charles F., *The Bubonic Plague and England* (University of Kentucky Press, 1956)

O'Donoghue, Edward Geoffrey, *Bridewell Hospital* (John Lane, 1929)

Parsons, F.G., *The History of St. Thomas's Hospital*, vol.II (Methuen, 1934)

Porter, Stephen, ed., *London and the Civil War* (Macmillan, 1996)

Porter, Stephen, *The Great Plague* (Sutton Publishing, 1999)

Rappaport, Steve, *Worlds within worlds: structures of life in sixteenth-century London* (Cambridge University Press, 1989)

Reed, Conyers, *Mr. Secretary Cecil and Queen Elizabeth* (Jonathan Cape, 1965)

Rosen, George, *A History of Public Health* (John Hopkins University Press, 1993)

Schen, Claire S., *Charity and Lay Piety in Reformation London, 1500–1620* (Ashgate, 2002)

Scott, Susan and Duncan, Christopher, *Biology of Plagues: Evidence from Historical Populations* (Cambridge University Press, 2001)

Seaver, Paul S., *Wallington's World: A Puritan Artisan in Seventeenth-Century London* (Methuen, 1985)

Sheppard, Francis, *London: A History* (Oxford University Press, 1998)

Shrewsbury, J.F.D., *The Plague of the Philistines and other Medico-Historical Essays* (Victor Gollancz, 1964)

—, *A History of Bubonic Plague in the British Isles* (Cambridge University Press, 1970)

Slack, Paul, *The Impact of Plague in Tudor and Stuart England* (Routledge & Kegan Paul, 1985)

—, *From reformation to improvement: public welfare in early modern England* (Oxford University Press, 1999)

Spicer, Andrew and Naphy, William, *Plague: Black Death & Pestilence in Europe* (Tempus Publishing, 2004)

The Survey of London, XIX, app.B (LCC, 1930)

Walsham, Alexandra, *Providence in Early Modern England* (Oxford University Press, 1999)

Wills, Christopher, *Plagues: Their Origins, History and Future* (HarperCollins, 1996)

Wilson, F.P., *The Plague in Shakespeare's London* (Oxford University Press, 1927, and later editions)

Woolley, Benjamin, *The Herbalist, Nicholas Culpeper and the Fight for Medical Freedom* (HarperCollins, 2004)

Wrigley, E.A. and Schofield, R.S., *The Population History of England 1541–1871* (Arnold, 1981)

Ziegler, Philip, *The Black Death* (Collins, 1969)

Articles

Achtman, Mark, *et al.*, 'Yersinia pestis, the cause of plague, is a recently emerged clone of Yersinia pseudotuberculosis', *Proc. of the National Academy of Sciences*, 96 (1999), 14043–8

Appleby, Andrew B., 'The Disappearance of Plague: A Continuing Puzzle', *Economic History Review*, XXXIII (1980), 161–73

Basing, Patricia and Rhodes, Dennis E., 'English plague regulations

and Italian models: printed and manuscript items in the Yelverton
collection', *British Library Journal*, 23 (1997), 60-7

Berry, Herbert, 'A London Plague Bill for 1592, Crick and Goodwyffe
Hurde', *English Literary Renaissance*, 25 (1995), 3-25

Caldin, Winefride and Raine, Helen, 'The plague of 1625 and the story
of John Boston, parish clerk of St Saviour's, Southwark', *Trans. of the
London and Middlesex Archaeological Soc.*, 23 (1971-2), 90-9

Cooper, William Durrant, 'Notices of the last Great Plague, 1665-6;
from the letters of John Allin to Philip Fryth and Samuel Jeake',
Archaeologia, 37 (1857), 1-22

Deng, Wen, *et al.*, 'Genome sequence of Yersinia pestis KIM', *Jnl of
Bacteriology*, 184 (2002), 4601-11

Gage, K.L., 'Plague' in Topley and Wilson's *Microbiology and microbial
infections*, 9th edn, ed. Leslie Collier *et al* (Arnold, 1998)

Grell, Ole Peter, 'Plague in Elizabethan and Stuart London: the Dutch
response', *Medical History*, 34 (1990), 424-39

Hollingsworth, Mary F. and Hollingsworth, T.H., 'Plague mortality rates
by age and sex in the parish of St Botolph's without Bishopsgate,
London, 1603', *Population Studies*, 25 (1971), 131-46

Jewers, Arthur J., 'The will of a plague-stricken Londoner', *Home Counties
Magazine*, 3 (1901), 109-10 [for Richard Lane]

Munkhoff, Richelle, 'Searchers of the Dead: Authority, Marginality, and
the Interpretation of Plague in England, 1574-1665', *Gender & History*,
11 (1999), 1-29

Munro, Ian, 'The City and its Double: Plague Time in Early Modern
London', *English Literary Renaissance*, 30 (2000), 241-61

Porter, Stephen, 'An historical whodunit', *The Biologist*, 51 (2004), 109-13

Poynter, F.N.L., 'A 17th century London plague document in the
Wellcome Historical Medical Library: Dr. Louis Du Moulin's
proposals to parliament for a corps of salaried plague-doctors', *Bulletin
of the History of Medicine*, 34 (1960), 365-72

Robertson, J.C., 'Reckoning with London: interpreting the Bills of
Mortality before John Graunt', *Urban History*, 23 (1996), 325-50

Slack, Paul, 'The Disappearance of Plague: An Alternative View', *Economic
History Review*, XXXIV (1981), 469-76

Sutherland, Ian, 'When was the Great Plague? Mortality in London, 1563
to 1665', in *Population and Social Change*, ed. D.V. Glass and Roger
Revelle (Arnold, 1972)

Symonds, E.M., 'The Diary of John Greene (1635–57)', *English Historical
Review*, XLIII (1928), XLIV (1929)

Wallis, Patrick, 'Plagues, Morality and the Place of Medicine in Early
Modern England', *English Historical Review*, CXXXI (2006), 1–24

List of Illustrations

to the church of St Mary Spital. Courtesy of Jonathan Reeve
JR854b46fp40 15501600.

10   To the west of the City, a ribbon-development of houses and
palaces led to Charing Cross, in the centre of this plan, and
continued to Westminster, with its abbey church and royal palace.
Tempus Archive TA CD 20, 189 15501600.

11   The Strand, between Ludgate, at the extreme right, and Durham
House, lined with aristocratic mansions and bishops' palaces.
Courtesy of Jonathan Reeve JR853b46fp22 15501600.

12   The Tower of London and Tower Wharf and, beyond them,
Whitechapel and East Smithfield. Courtesy of Jonathan Reeve JR
CD31025 15501600.

13   The Tower *c.*1597. Tempus Archive TA CD 20,173 15501600.

14   The Black Death reached England in 1348, during the reign of
Edward III. In this drawing of a wall painting in St Stephen's
chapel, Westminster, the king and St George are shown praying.
Courtesy of Jonathan Reeve JR719b18p204 13001350.

15   The Black Death may have killed as much as one-third of the
population, producing a serious shortage of labour, and so the
opportunity for improved conditions. The government attempted
to curb this by the Ordinance of Labourers of 1349, shown here.
Courtesy of Jonathan Reeve JR725b13p487 13001350.

16   Plague was a disease spread along the trade routes and an added
danger for sailors. Holbein shows a ship battered in a storm, with
Death clinging to the broken mast. Tempus Archive.

17   London was a major seaport; Wyngaerde's view shows shipping on
the Thames downstream from London. Tempus Archive TA CD
20, 104 15501600.

18   Customs dues on goods landed at London were paid at the
Custom House. Tempus Archive TA CD 20 216 15501600.

19   In Holbein's *Dance of Death* series, a merchant is eager to check
his bales of newly landed goods, but Death is already plucking at
his cloak. Tempus Archive.

20   Henry VIII painted by Hans Holbein. Tempus Archive TA CD 12,
25.

21   Following the destruction of the royal living quarters at
Westminster Palace by fire in 1512, Bridewell Palace was adapted
as the king's residence in London. By 1660 it had become a
prison. Tempus Archive TA CD 20, 186 16501700.

22   Henry VIII began the development of York Place as the royal
palace of Whitehall, shown only sketchily by Wyngaerde, alongside
the Thames between Westminster, with its abbey and St Stephen's
church, and Durham House, close to the right of the drawing.

Courtesy of Jonathan Reeve JR729b46fp16 13001350.

23 A model of the plague doctor in the Museum de
    Stratemakerstoren in Nijmegen. Author's Collection.

24 Holbein shows that a nobleman's weapons were futile against
    the plague, for Death pulls at him as his life, measured by the
    hourglass, is ebbing away and his coffin awaits. Tempus Archive.

25 Holbein develops a similar theme in 'Death and the Count', as
    Death takes away the count's armour, leaving him defenceless.
    Tempus Archive.

26 In a scene from the *Dance of Death*, an abbot is pulled away by the
    skeletal figure of Death masquerading as a bishop. Tempus Archive.

27 Even a poor friar, collecting alms and carrying his food, cannot escape
    Death, which pulls him back as he attempts to flee. Tempus Archive.

28 A nun, carrying her rosary, is taken from her convent by Death, to
    the horror of her fellow nun. Tempus Archive.

29 A section of the plan-view of London in Georg Braun and Frans
    Hogenberg's *Civitatis Orbis Terrarum* (1572), with St Paul's at the
    centre. Tempus Archive TA46b51fp432 15501600.

30 The leading citizens were responsible for enforcing the plague
    regulations. Holbein shows the town notables completing a
    transaction, but Death, with his hourglass, stands by listening to
    their conversation. Tempus Archive.

31 In this woodcut from *A Looking-glasse for City and Countrey*
    (1630) citizens flee London by coach, on horseback and on foot,
    yet Death, with spear and hourglass, stalks them, and has already
    claimed a victim. Tempus Archive.

32 Some who fled from plague in London went to nearby villages,
    such as Islington, shown here on a mid-sixteenth-century plan.
    Tempus Archive TA CD 20, 193 15501600.

33 Death leads this bishop away through the fields. The people are
    distraught as their spiritual shepherd is taken from them, while the
    sheep look on. Tempus Archive.

34 Plague burials were conducted at night, so Death carries a lantern.
    Tempus Archive.

35 The magistrates oversaw the maintenance of law and order and
    the administration of the government's plague policies, but even
    as the judge is speaking, Death is reaching out for him. Tempus
    Archive.

36 Thomas White condemned plays as a cause of plague in a sermon
    in 1577. During plague outbreaks the authorities disapproved
    of such gatherings, but their orders were difficult to enforce, as
    Londoners continued to attend services. Courtesy of Jonathan
    Reeve JR209b5068 15501600.

51 Wenceslaus Hollar's drawing shows a length of the New River in
    Islington. Tempus Archive TA23b50plaxliv 16001650.

52 Plan of parts of the parishes of St Martin Outwich, to the left, and
    St Peter's, Cornhill, drawn in 1599. Tempus Archive TA CD 20
    192, 15501600.

53 The procession bringing Charles I's mother-in-law, Marie
    de Medici, to London in 1638. Courtesy of Jonathan Reeve
    JR445b8fp94 16001650.

54 The riverfront running eastwards from the Savoy to the Temple,
    with its gardens. Courtesy of Jonathan Reeve JR269b10p1073
    16001650.

55 Four-storey houses in Leadenhall Street, with jettied upper floors
    overhanging the street. Courtesy of Jonathan Reeve JR855b8fp54
    15501600.

56 New Palace Yard, with Westminster Hall and the Clock House,
    an engraving by Wenceslaus Hollar, 1647. Tempus Archive
    TA30b50plali 166001650.

57 Westminster from the river, by Hollar, 1647. Courtesy of Jonathan
    Reeve JR274b10p1116 16001650.

58 Hollar's plan of mid-seventeenth-century London shows the
    extent to which the city had expanded. Crown copyright,
    NMR.

59 Hollar's Long View of London from Southwark, 1647, depicts
    a city which had grown to be the second largest in northern
    Europe, after Paris. Tempus Archive.

60 Hollar chose a different perspective in this later view across the
    Thames from Lambeth. Tempus Archive TA7b50plaix 16001650.

61 The narrow streets and tall buildings around Smithfield c.1900.
    Crown copyright, NMR.

62 Peter's Lane, Clerkenwell, c.1900, on the north side of Smithfield.
    Crown copyright, NMR.

63 The parish of St Giles-in-the Fields in 1570. Tempus Archive.

64 St Giles-in-the Fields was in an area with much poor housing,
    but also wealthy neighbourhoods, such as Lincoln's Inn Fields,
    developed in the late 1630s and shown here on Hollar's engraving
    of c.1657. Tempus Archive TA24b50plaxlvi 16001650.

65 The Piazza in Covent Garden, with St Paul's church, drawn by
    Hollar. Tempus Archive TA25b50plaxlvii 16001650.

66 The disease has struck this relatively well-to-do family, with the
    sick being nursed in their beds and a member of the household
    laid on the floor, close to a coffin. Courtesy of William Naphy
    and Andrew Spicer.

67 This street scene illustrating the Great Plague has many of the

with 4,237 of the total of 5,568 attributed to plague. Courtesy of William Naphy and Andrew Spicer.

82   The figures for the year were published in a collection and summary of the Bills of Mortality, expressively entitled *London's Dreadful Visitation*. Author's Collection.

83   The summary of the Bills for 1665 shows the numbers buried and those deaths attributed to plague, by parish, and the total numbers by cause of death. Author's Collection.

84   As the number of plague deaths recorded in the Bills declined, those who had left London steadily returned to the city. Courtesy of William Naphy and Andrew Spicer.

85   Southwark suffered badly in the Great Plague; the crowded buildings there were shown on Hollar's engraving of 1647. Crown copyright, NMR.

86   The Great Plague was followed in September 1666 by the Great Fire of London. Courtesy of Jonathan Reeve JR856b8fp84 15501600.

87   The title page of *A Journal of the Plague Year* by Daniel Defoe. Author's Collection.

Index

TEMPUS – REVEALING HISTORY

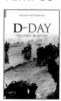 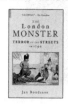

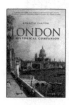

D-Day The First 72 Hours
WILLIAM F. BUCKINGHAM

'A compelling narrative' *The Observer*

A *BBC History Magazine* Book of the Year 2004

£9.99   0 7524 2842 X

The London Monster
Terror on the Streets in 1790

JAN BONDESON

'Gripping' *The Guardian*

'Excellent... monster-mania brought a reign of terror to the ill-lit streets of the capital' *The Independent*

£9.99   0 7524 3327 X

London
A Historical Companion

KENNETH PANTON

'A readable and reliable work of reference that deserves a place on every Londoner's bookshelf' *Stephen Inwood*

£20   0 7524 3434 9

M: MI5's First Spymaster
ANDREW COOK

'Serious spook history' *Andrew Roberts*

'Groundbreaking' *The Sunday Telegraph*

'Brilliantly researched' *Dame Stella Rimington*

£9.99   978 07524 3949 9

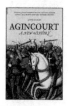 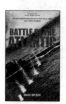

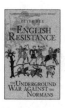 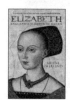

Agincourt
A New History

ANNE CURRY

'A highly distinguished and convincing account' *Christopher Hibbert*

'A *tour de force*' *Alison Weir*

'*The* book on the battle' *Richard Holmes*

A *BBC History Magazine* Book of the Year 2005

£12.99   0 7524 3813 1

Battle of the Atlantic
MARC MILNER

'The most comprehensive short survey of the U-boat battles' *Sir John Keegan*

'Some events are fortunate in their historian, none more so than the Battle of the Atlantic. Marc Milner is *the* historian of the Atlantic campaign... a compelling narrative' *Andrew Lambert*

£12.99   0 7524 3332 6

The English Resistance
The Underground War Against the Normans

PETER REX

'An invaluable rehabilitation of an ignored resistance movement' *The Sunday Times*

'Peter Rex's scholarship is remarkable' *The Sunday Express*

£12.99   0 7524 3733 X

Elizabeth Wydeville: England's Slandered Queen
ARLENE OKERLUND

'A penetrating, thorough and wholly convincing vindication of this unlucky queen' *Sarah Gristwood*

'A gripping tale of lust, loss and tragedy' *Alison Weir*

A *BBC History Magazine* Book of the Year 2005

£9.99   978 07524 3807 8

If you are interested in purchasing other books published by Tempus, or in case you have difficulty finding any Tempus books in your local bookshop, you can also place orders directly through our website

www.tempus-publishing.com

TEMPUS – REVEALING HISTORY

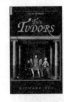
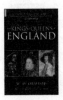

Quacks Fakers and Charlatans in Medicine
ROY PORTER

'A delightful book' *The Daily Telegraph*
'Hugely entertaining' *BBC History Magazine*

£12.99   0 7524 2590 0

The Tudors
RICHARD REX

'Up-to-date, readable and reliable. The best introduction to England's most important dynasty' *David Starkey*
'Vivid, entertaining... quite simply the best short introduction' *Eamon Duffy*
'Told with enviable narrative skill... a delight for any reader' *THES*

£9.99   0 7524 3333 4

The Kings & Queens of England
MARK ORMROD

'Of the numerous books on the kings and queens of England, this is the best'
Alison Weir

£9.99   0 7524 2598 6

The Covent Garden Ladies
Pimp General Jack & the Extraordinary Story of Harris's List
HALLIE RUBENHOLD

'Sex toys, porn... forget Ann Summers, Miss Love was at it 250 years ago' *The Times*
'Compelling' *The Independent on Sunday*
'Marvellous' *Leonie Frieda*
'Filthy' *The Guardian*

£9.99   0 7524 3739 9

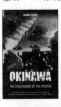
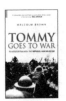

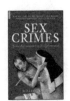

Okinawa 1945
GEORGE FEIFER

'A great book... Feifer's account of the three sides and their experiences far surpasses most books about war'
Stephen Ambrose

£17.99   0 7524 3324 5

Tommy Goes To War
MALCOLM BROWN

'A remarkably vivid and frank account of the British soldier in the trenches'
Max Arthur
'The fury, fear, mud, blood, boredom and bravery that made up life on the Western Front are vividly presented and illustrated'
The Sunday Telegraph

£12.99   0 7524 2980 4

Ace of Spies The True Story of Sidney Reilly
ANDREW COOK

'The most definitive biography of the spying ace yet written... both a compelling narrative and a myth-shattering *tour de force*'
Simon Sebag Montefiore
'The absolute last word on the subject' *Nigel West*
'Makes poor 007 look like a bit of a wuss'
The Mail on Sunday

£12.99   0 7524 2959 0

Sex Crimes
From Renaissance to Enlightenment
W.M. NAPHY

'Wonderfully scandalous' *Diarmaid MacCulloch*
'A model of pin-sharp scholarship' *The Guardian*

£10.99   0 7524 2977 9